RURAL GENERAL EMERGENCY POCKET GUIDE

DR. MOHAMED ELGENDY
LMCC, CCFP CANADA

DISCLAIMER

This pocket guide was developed with the assistance of advanced AI tools to streamline content generation. Every chapter has been thoroughly reviewed, edited, and authenticated by Dr. Mohamed Elgendy, LMCC, CCFP (Canada), ensuring accuracy, credibility, and clinical authenticity. The result is a modern, innovative reference that blends the efficiency of AI with the rigor of professional medical expertise.

This pocket guide summarizes common emergency medicine and rural ER approaches using only open-access guidance; no proprietary or subscription-based content is reproduced.

Clinical descriptions (including assessments, investigations, and treatments) are abbreviated for educational purposes and exam preparation. They are not intended as complete protocols or substitutes for independent clinical judgment.

Management should always be performed within the clinician's scope of training, local regulations, and available resources, with appropriate patient consent, monitoring, and safety measures. Escalate care promptly when red flags arise (e.g., airway compromise, hemodynamic instability, severe infection, suspected surgical emergency, or complex multi-morbidity) or when the situation exceeds your competence or resources.

Always confirm current local and national guidelines, product monographs/labels, and institutional pathways before application. Verify patient-specific contraindications, comorbidities, and drug interactions. Clinical responsibility remains with the treating clinician.

DEDICATION

This guide is dedicated to the patients in rural and remote communities—whose resilience and courage inspire every clinical decision; to the clinicians, nurses, medics, and allied staff who deliver essential emergency care with skill and compassion despite distance, resource limitations, and isolation; to mentors and colleagues who freely share knowledge so that care remains safe and evidence-informed; and to my family, whose unwavering support sustains this work.

May this concise, open-access emergency pocket guide serve them all.

— Dr. Mohamed Elgendy

ABOUT THE AUTHIOR

Dr. Mohamed Elgendy is a licensed Canadian physician with the Licentiate of the Medical Council of Canada (LMCC) and Certification in Family Medicine (CCFP) from the College of Family Physicians of Canada.

He has extensive hands-on experience as both a rural emergency physician and family doctor, currently practicing in Saskatchewan, Canada. With a deep commitment to improving emergency and acute care in underserved communities, Dr. Elgendy focuses on practical, evidence-based emergency medicine adapted to the realities of rural practice.

His work bridges the gap between academic guidelines and frontline clinical realities, offering accessible, concise resources to help clinicians make confident, lifesaving decisions in resource-limited settings.

INDEX — CATEGORIZED

- DISCLAIMER.. iii

- DEDICATION.. v

- ABOUT THE AUTHIOR.. vii

- Procedures Index — Categorized ix

SECTION I – GENERAL PRINCIPLES 1

- Initial Emergency Assessment (ABCD in Rural Settings)...................... 2

- Stabilization and Transport Considerations.......................... 4

- Pain Management and Procedural Sedation in Limited-Resource Settings.................... 6

SECTION II – CARDIOVASCULAR EMERGENCIES 8

- Chest Pain: STEMI, NSTEMI, Unstable Angina — Rural ER Approach.. 9

- Arrhythmias (AFib, SVT, VT/VF, Bradycardia) — Rural ER Approach.. 14

- Hypertensive Emergencies vs Urgencies — Rural ER Approach........ 19

- Heart Failure and Acute Pulmonary Edema — Rural ER Approach ... 24

- Cardiac Arrest & ACLS Algorithms — Rural ER Approach.................. 29

SECTION III – RESPIRATORY EMERGENCIES 34

- Acute Asthma Exacerbation — Rural ER Approach 35

- COPD Exacerbation — Rural ER Approach 40

- Pneumonia in Adults & Children (Community-Acquired Pneumonia, CAP) — Rural ER Approach 45

- Anaphylaxis (Recognition & Epinephrine Dosing) — Rural ER Approach... 50

- Upper Airway Emergencies (Epiglottitis, Foreign Body, Angioedema) —

Rural ER Approach 55

* Respiratory Distress in Infants (Bronchiolitis, Croup) — Rural ER
  Approach 60

SECTION IV –NEUROLOGICAL EMERGENCIES 65

* Acute Stroke (Recognition, tPA/Transfer Criteria) —
  Rural ER Approach 66

* Seizures and Status Epilepticus — Rural ER Approach 71

* Head Injury (Adult & Pediatric Concussion/Trauma) —
  Rural ER Approach 76

* Dizziness & Vertigo (Central vs Peripheral Red Flags) —
  Rural ER Approach 83

SECTION V – ABDOMINAL & GASTROINTESTINAL EMERGENCIES 90

* Acute Abdominal Pain (Red Flags in Rural ER) —
  Rural ER Approach 91

* Gastrointestinal Bleeding (Upper vs Lower) —
  Rural ER Approach 97

* Bowel Obstruction & Perforation Suspicion —
  Rural ER Approach 102

* Pediatric Abdominal Emergencies (Appendicitis, Intussusception) —
  Rural ER Approach 107

SECTION VI – RENAL & UROLOGIC EMERGENCIES... 112

* Renal Colic & Kidney Stones — Rural ER Approach 113

* Hyperkalemia & Hypokalemia (Rural ER Approach) 118

* Electrolyte Disturbances — Hypercalcemia & Hypocalcemia
  (Rural ER Approach) 123

* Electrolyte Disturbances — Hyponatremia & Hypernatremia
  (Rural ER Approach) 128

SECTION VII – INFECTIOUS DISEASES 133

* Sepsis Recognition & Management — Rural ER Approach 134

* Meningitis & Encephalitis (Empiric Antibiotics) —

Rural ER Approach 139

◆ Fever in the Returning Traveler (Malaria, Dengue, etc.) —
  Rural ER Approach.. 144

◆ Common Rural Outbreaks (Influenza, Gastroenteritis, COVID, TB Basics)
  — Rural ER Approach 150

◆ Tuberculosis (TB) — Rural ER Basics 155

◆ COVID-19 — Rural ER Approach 161

◆ Gastroenteritis — Rural ER Approach 165

◆ Influenza — Rural ER Approach.. 170

◆ Skin & Soft Tissue Infections (Cellulitis, Erysipelas, Abscess, MRSA,
  Necrotizing Fasciitis) — Rural ER Approach...................................... 175

SECTION VIII – ONCOLOGIC EMERGENCIES 180

◆ Oncologic Emergencies — Rural ER Approach 181

◆ Spinal Cord Compression — Rural ER Approach 187

◆ Superior Vena Cava (SVC) Syndrome — Rural ER Approach............ 192

◆ Febrile Neutropenia — Rural ER Approach 197

SECTION IX –TRAUMA AND ORTHOPEDIC 202

◆ Common Fractures & Dislocations (Initial Splinting, Transfer Criteria) —
  Rural ER Approach.. 203

◆ Compartment Syndrome (Recognition & Action) —
  Rural ER Approach.. 208

◆ Wound Management (Closure, Tetanus, Antibiotics for Bites/Open
  Wounds) — Rural ER Approach... 212

SECTION X – PEDIATRICS 217

◆ Pediatric Fever (Neonate vs Child) — Rural ER Approach 218

◆ Pediatric Respiratory Distress (Asthma, Bronchiolitis, Croup) —
  Rural ER Approach.. 223

◆ Pediatric Seizures & Febrile Seizures — Rural ER Approach............ 228

SECTION XI – OBSTETRICS & GYNECOLOGY 234

- Early Pregnancy Emergencies (Ectopic, Miscarriage) — Rural ER Approach 235

- Third-Trimester Emergencies (Pre-eclampsia, Eclampsia, Placental Abruption) — Rural ER Approach 240

- Normal Delivery in the ER (Precipitous Birth, Shoulder Dystocia, Postpartum Hemorrhage) — Rural ER Approach 246

- Vaginal Bleeding & Vaginitis — Rural ER Approach 251

SECTION I –
GENERAL PRINCIPLES

INITIAL EMERGENCY ASSESSMENT (ABCD IN RURAL SETTINGS)

OVERVIEW:

Initial emergency assessment follows the Airway, Breathing, Circulation, Disability (ABCD) framework. In rural settings, clinicians often face limited staff, equipment, and delayed access to advanced imaging or specialist support. Rapid assessment is critical to stabilize life-threatening conditions early.

MANAGEMENT IN RURAL ER (WITH DRUG DOSES)

1. Airway: Ensure patency, suction secretions, insert oropharyngeal airway (OPA) or nasopharyngeal airway (NPA). If intubation is required and trained staff are available: Etomidate 0.3 mg/kg IV or Ketamine 1–2 mg/kg IV for induction; Succinylcholine 1–1.5 mg/kg IV or Rocuronium 1.2 mg/kg IV for paralysis.
2. Breathing: Oxygen 10–15 L/min via non-rebreather mask. Bag-valve-mask ventilation if inadequate

respiration. Nebulized salbutamol 2.5–5 mg q20min PRN for bronchospasm.

3. Circulation: Establish IV/IO access. IV fluids: Normal saline or Ringer's lactate bolus 500–1000 mL in adults, 20 mL/kg in pediatrics. If shock persists, consider epinephrine infusion (2–10 mcg/min IV) or norepinephrine (2–20 mcg/min IV titrated to MAP >65 mmHg).

4. Disability: Check glucose; if hypoglycemia → Dextrose 25 g IV (D50W 50 mL). In pediatrics, D10W 5 mL/kg IV. Seizure control: Diazepam 5–10 mg IV q10–15min PRN (max 30 mg) or Lorazepam 4 mg IV at 2 mg/min, may repeat once.

STABILIZATION AND TRANSPORT CONSIDERATIONS

OVERVIEW:

In rural practice, transport to tertiary centers is often required for definitive care. Stabilization prior to transfer ensures patient safety during prolonged travel by ground or air.

CLINICAL PRIORITIES AND MEDICATIONS

1. Secure airway before transfer if high risk of deterioration (use RSI drugs as above if needed).
2. Oxygen therapy as required.
3. Establish 2 large-bore IVs. If shock present: start IV fluids (500–1000 mL NS bolus; pediatric 20 mL/kg). Add vasopressors if no response (Norepinephrine 2–20 mcg/min IV titrated; Dopamine 5–20 mcg/kg/min IV infusion).
4. Adequate analgesia: Morphine 2–5 mg IV q5–10min PRN (max 10 mg); Fentanyl 25–50 mcg IV q5min PRN.
5. Sedation if intubated: Midazolam 2–5 mg IV q5–10min

PRN or infusion 0.02–0.1 mg/kg/hr.

6. Control bleeding: TXA (tranexamic acid) 1 g IV over 10 min, followed by 1 g IV over 8 hrs if trauma with major bleeding.

PAIN MANAGEMENT AND PROCEDURAL SEDATION IN LIMITED-RESOURCE SETTINGS

OVERVIEW:

Pain control is an essential component of emergency care. In rural ERs, limited drug formulary and monitoring capabilities make safe choices and proper dosing critical. Procedural sedation should be used judiciously when transfer delays definitive care.

ANALGESIA AND SEDATION (WITH DRUG DOSES)

Non-Pharmacological:
1. Splinting, positioning, reassurance, distraction techniques.

Pharmacological:
1. Acetaminophen: Adults 650–1000 mg PO/IV q6h (max 4 g/day); Pediatrics 15 mg/kg PO/IV q6h (max 75 mg/kg/day).

2. Ibuprofen: Adults 400–600 mg PO q6–8h (max 2400 mg/day); Pediatrics 10 mg/kg PO q6–8h (max 40 mg/kg/day).

3. Morphine: Adults 2–5 mg IV q5–10min PRN (max 10 mg); Pediatrics 0.1 mg/kg IV q2–4h.

4. Fentanyl: Adults 25–50 mcg IV q5min PRN (max 200 mcg/hr); Pediatrics 1 mcg/kg IV q1–2h.

Procedural Sedation:

1. Ketamine: 1–2 mg/kg IV over 1 min OR 4–5 mg/kg IM. Provides analgesia and sedation while preserving airway reflexes.

2. Midazolam: Adults 2–5 mg IV slow push; Pediatrics 0.1 mg/kg IV (max 2–3 mg).

3. Fentanyl: 25–50 mcg IV for adjunctive analgesia.

4. Always monitor SpO_2, HR, BP, and be prepared for airway management (BVM, suction, intubation backup).

REFERENCES

1. Emergency Care BC – https://emergencycarebc.ca/clinical_resource

2. Heart & Stroke Foundation of Canada – https://cpr.heartandstroke.ca

3. Canadian Paediatric Society – https://cps.ca

4. Thrombosis Canada – https://thrombosiscanada.ca

5. CDC Emergency Preparedness – https://www.cdc.gov

6. WHO Emergency Care Guidance – https://www.who.int

SECTION II – CARDIOVASCULAR EMERGENCIES

CHEST PAIN: STEMI, NSTEMI, UNSTABLE ANGINA — RURAL ER APPROACH

OVERVIEW

Acute Coronary Syndrome (ACS) includes ST-Elevation Myocardial Infarction (STEMI),

Non-ST Elevation Myocardial Infarction (NSTEMI), and Unstable Angina (UA). Early recognition and treatment are critical to improve survival. Rural emergency physicians face challenges with limited diagnostics and lack of immediate PCI. Management focuses on stabilization, thrombolysis (if PCI unavailable), and transfer.

CLINICAL PRESENTATION

1. Classic: central chest pain/pressure radiating to arm, neck, or jaw.
2. Associated: diaphoresis, nausea, vomiting, shortness of breath, syncope.
3. Atypical: fatigue, dyspnea, confusion, abdominal pain — more common in elderly, women, diabetics.

9

RED FLAGS

1. Hemodynamic instability (hypotension, shock).
2. Ongoing chest pain despite nitroglycerin.
3. Arrhythmias (VT/VF, severe bradycardia).
4. New heart failure or pulmonary edema.
5. ST elevation or new LBBB on ECG.

DIFFERENTIAL DIAGNOSIS

1. Pulmonary embolism.
2. Aortic dissection.
3. Pneumothorax.
4. Pericarditis.
5. GI causes: reflux, esophageal spasm.

INVESTIGATIONS

1. ECG: within 10 minutes of arrival, repeat if nondiagnostic.
2. Bedside: vitals, SpO_2, glucose.
3. Labs (if available): troponin, CBC, electrolytes, creatinine.
4. Chest X-ray: to exclude other causes (should not delay treatment).

MANAGEMENT IN RURAL ER (WITH DRUG DOSAGES)

Immediate stabilization:

1. Oxygen if $SpO_2 < 90\%$.

2. IV access ×2, continuous monitoring.

3. Aspirin 160–325 mg PO chewed immediately.

4. Nitroglycerin 0.4 mg SL q5min ×3 max if SBP > 100 mmHg (avoid if RV infarct or PDE-5 inhibitor use).

5. Morphine 2–5 mg IV q5–10min PRN (max 10 mg) if pain persists.

STEMI:

1. If PCI <120 min available → transfer for PCI.

2. If PCI unavailable → Fibrinolysis (Tenecteplase IV single bolus: <60 kg = 30 mg; 60–69 kg = 35 mg; 70–79 kg = 40 mg; "

"80–89 kg = 45 mg; ≥90 kg = 50 mg).

1. Adjunct: Clopidogrel 300 mg PO load (<75 yr) then 75 mg daily; ≥75 yr no load.

2. Anticoagulation: Enoxaparin 30 mg IV bolus then 1 mg/kg SC q12h (<75 yr); ≥75 yr omit IV bolus, use 0.75 mg/kg SC q12h.

NSTEMI/UA:

1. ASA as above.

2. Clopidogrel 300 mg PO load (<75 yr) then 75 mg daily.

3. Anticoagulation: Enoxaparin 1 mg/kg SC q12h.

4. Rate control if AFib: Metoprolol 5 mg IV q5min ×3 (hold if hypotension or CHF).

5. Nitrates and morphine for symptom relief.

6. Transfer for cardiology evaluation.

WHEN TO CALL A SPECIALIST / TRANSFER

1. All suspected ACS require cardiology consultation.
2. STEMI → immediate PCI transfer or fibrinolysis if PCI unavailable.
3. NSTEMI/UA with high-risk features → transfer for early intervention.
4. Unstable patients requiring advanced support.

DISPOSITION

1. Discharge: rare, only if ACS ruled out with serial ECG/troponins and low risk.
2. Admit locally: if stable but awaiting transfer.
3. Transfer: most ACS patients should be transferred to higher-level facility.

ADMISSION ORDERS (RURAL HOSPITAL)

1. Admit to monitored bed if available.
2. Oxygen if hypoxemic.
3. ASA 81 mg PO daily after loading dose.
4. Clopidogrel 75 mg PO daily after loading.
5. Enoxaparin per weight and age protocol.
6. Beta-blocker: Metoprolol PO 25–50 mg q12h if stable.
7. Nitroglycerin infusion: 5 mcg/min IV, titrate q5min by 5 mcg/min up to 20 mcg/min (max 200 mcg/min).
8. Pain: Morphine 2–5 mg IV q5–10min PRN.

REFERENCES

1. Heart & Stroke Foundation of Canada – https://cpr. heartandstroke.ca
2. Emergency Care BC – https://emergencycarebc.ca/ clinical_resource
3. Thrombosis Canada – https://thrombosiscanada.ca
4. Canadian Cardiovascular Society – https://ccs.ca
5. CDC – https://www.cdc.gov/heartdisease/heart_attack. htm

ARRHYTHMIAS (AFIB, SVT, VT/ VF, BRADYCARDIA) — RURAL ER APPROACH

OVERVIEW

Arrhythmias range from benign to immediately life-threatening. In rural ERs, rapid recognition and stabilization are essential, especially when advanced monitoring and cardiology support may not be readily available. Management focuses on distinguishing unstable vs stable rhythms and initiating appropriate drug or electrical therapy while arranging transfer.

CLINICAL PRESENTATION

1. Atrial Fibrillation (AFib): palpitations, irregular pulse, fatigue, dizziness, chest discomfort, possible heart failure.
2. Supraventricular Tachycardia (SVT): sudden palpitations, lightheadedness, chest pain, may terminate spontaneously.

3. Ventricular Tachycardia (VT): palpitations, chest pain, syncope, dyspnea; may progress to VF.

4. Ventricular Fibrillation (VF): pulseless cardiac arrest, unresponsive.

5. Bradycardia: dizziness, syncope, fatigue, hypotension, possible asystole.

RED FLAGS

1. Hemodynamic instability: hypotension, chest pain, altered mental status, shock.

2. Wide complex tachycardia (treat as VT until proven otherwise).

3. Bradycardia with hypotension not responding to atropine.

4. Cardiac arrest rhythms: VF, pulseless VT.

DIFFERENTIAL DIAGNOSIS

1. Electrolyte abnormalities (K+, Mg++, Ca++).

2. Thyroid disease (hyperthyroidism in AFib).

3. Drug toxicity (digoxin, beta-blockers, calcium channel blockers).

4. Hypoxia, sepsis, ACS.

5. Anxiety, benign palpitations.

INVESTIGATIONS

1. ECG: rhythm, rate, QRS width, ischemic changes.

2. Bedside: vitals, SpO_2, glucose.

3. Labs (if available): CBC, electrolytes, creatinine,

troponin, thyroid function if new AFib.

4.   Chest X-ray: if heart failure suspected.

MANAGEMENT IN RURAL ER (WITH DRUG DOSAGES)

Atrial Fibrillation (AFib):

1.   Unstable (hypotension, chest pain, shock): synchronized cardioversion starting at 100 J (biphasic).

2.   Stable: rate control — Metoprolol 5 mg IV q5min ×3 (max 15 mg), then PO 25–50 mg q6–12h; or Diltiazem 0.25 mg/kg IV over 2 min, may repeat 0.35 mg/kg after 15 min, then infusion 5–15 mg/hr.

3.   Anticoagulation: Enoxaparin 1 mg/kg SC q12h.

Supraventricular Tachycardia (SVT):

1.   Vagal maneuvers first.

2.   Adenosine 6 mg IV rapid bolus; if no response, 12 mg IV. May repeat 12 mg once (max 30 mg).

3.   If unstable: synchronized cardioversion at 50–100 J.

Ventricular Tachycardia (VT):

1.   Pulseless: treat as VF — CPR, defibrillation 200 J biphasic, Epinephrine 1 mg IV q3–5min, Amiodarone 300 mg IV push, repeat 150 mg if needed.

2.   With pulse but unstable: synchronized cardioversion 100 J, increase as needed.

3. Stable monomorphic VT: Amiodarone 150 mg IV over 10 min, repeat as needed, then infusion 1 mg/min ×6h.

Ventricular Fibrillation (VF):

1. Immediate CPR and defibrillation (200 J biphasic).
2. Epinephrine 1 mg IV q3–5min.
3. Amiodarone 300 mg IV push, then 150 mg if recurrent.

Bradycardia:

1. Unstable: Atropine 0.5 mg IV q3–5min (max 3 mg).
2. If ineffective: transcutaneous pacing if available.
3. Dopamine infusion 5–20 mcg/kg/min IV or Epinephrine infusion 2–10 mcg/min IV if pacing unavailable.

WHEN TO CALL A SPECIALIST / TRANSFER

1. All unstable arrhythmias requiring cardioversion or defibrillation.
2. New-onset AFib with ACS, VT, VF.
3. Symptomatic bradycardia requiring pacing.
4. Any arrhythmia not controlled with initial therapy.
5. Early contact for transfer planning is essential.

DISPOSITION

1. Admit locally only if stable and monitoring available.
2. Transfer: most patients with significant arrhythmias

should be transferred for cardiology evaluation.

3. Discharge: rare, only after self-limited SVT or AFib with clear reversible trigger and reliable follow-up.

ADMISSION ORDERS (RURAL HOSPITAL)

1. Admit to monitored bed.
2. Continuous ECG monitoring.
3. Maintain IV access.
4. Oxygen as required.
5. Rhythm-specific medications (e.g., Metoprolol, Amiodarone, Enoxaparin).
6. Prepare for transfer if deterioration occurs.

REFERENCES

1. Heart & Stroke Foundation of Canada – https://cpr. heartandstroke.ca
2. Emergency Care BC – https://emergencycarebc.ca/ clinical_resource
3. Thrombosis Canada – https://thrombosiscanada. ca
4. Canadian Cardiovascular Society – https://ccs.ca
5. CDC – https://www.cdc.gov/heartdisease

HYPERTENSIVE EMERGENCIES VS URGENCIES — RURAL ER APPROACH

OVERVIEW

Hypertension is a common finding in the ER. Hypertensive emergency is defined as severe blood pressure elevation with acute target organ damage (e.g., stroke, ACS, pulmonary edema, renal failure, aortic dissection). Hypertensive urgency involves markedly elevated blood pressure without evidence of acute organ injury. Differentiating the two guides treatment.

CLINICAL PRESENTATION

Hypertensive Emergency:
1. Neurological: headache, confusion, visual changes, seizures, stroke.
2. Cardiac: chest pain, ACS, pulmonary edema.
3. Renal: oliguria, hematuria, rising creatinine.
4. Vascular: tearing chest/back pain (aortic dissection).

Hypertensive Urgency:

1. Severe BP elevation (often >180/110 mmHg).

2. Usually asymptomatic, sometimes mild headache or anxiety.

3. No acute organ dysfunction.

RED FLAGS

1. Neurological deficit (ischemic or hemorrhagic stroke).

2. Chest pain with dissection or ACS.

3. Pulmonary edema, heart failure.

4. Oliguria/renal failure.

5. Pregnancy-related hypertension (eclampsia, HELLP).

DIFFERENTIAL DIAGNOSIS

1. Anxiety, pain, or missed medications.

2. Stroke (ischemic/hemorrhagic).

3. Pheochromocytoma crisis.

4. Drug toxicity (cocaine, amphetamines).

5. Pregnancy: pre-eclampsia/eclampsia.

INVESTIGATIONS

1. Confirm BP in both arms, proper cuff size.

2. ECG: ischemia, arrhythmia, LVH.

3. Labs: electrolytes, creatinine, troponin, CBC, urinalysis.

4. Glucose bedside.

5. CXR: pulmonary edema, widened mediastinum.

6. CT head if neurological symptoms.

7. Pregnancy test in women of childbearing age.

MANAGEMENT IN RURAL ER (WITH DRUG DOSAGES)

Hypertensive Emergency:

1. Goal: lower MAP by max 25% in first hour.

2. Avoid rapid normalization to prevent ischemia.

IV Medications (if available):

1. Labetalol: 20 mg IV over 2 min, then 40–80 mg q10min PRN (max 300 mg) or infusion 2 mg/min.

2. Hydralazine: 5–10 mg IV q20–30min (esp. in pregnancy).

3. Nitroglycerin infusion: start 5 mcg/min, titrate by 5 mcg/min q5min (max 200 mcg/min).

4. Nitroprusside (if available): start 0.3 mcg/kg/min, titrate up to 10 mcg/kg/min (rare in rural sites).

Hypertensive Urgency:

1. No IV therapy required.

2. Start/adjust oral meds, gradual reduction over 24–48h.

Options:

1. Amlodipine 5–10 mg PO once daily.

2. Captopril 25 mg PO q8h.

3. Labetalol 100–200 mg PO q8–12h.

4. Clonidine 0.1–0.2 mg PO, may repeat in 1–2h (max 0.6 mg).

WHEN TO CALL A SPECIALIST / TRANSFER

1. All hypertensive emergencies (stroke, ACS, aortic dissection, pulmonary edema, pregnancy-related).
2. When IV antihypertensives unavailable or ineffective.
3. Early consultation improves outcomes.

DISPOSITION

1. Emergency: stabilize and transfer urgently.
2. Urgency: safe discharge with close follow-up and oral medication adjustment.
3. Admit locally if follow-up not feasible or social supports lacking.

ADMISSION ORDERS (RURAL HOSPITAL)

1. Admit to monitored bed if available.
2. Frequent BP and neuro checks.
3. IV access.
4. Start antihypertensives per severity.
5. Monitor urine output, electrolytes.
6. Prepare for transfer if emergency.

REFERENCES

1. Heart & Stroke Foundation of Canada – https://cpr. heartandstroke.ca

2. Emergency Care BC – https://emergencycarebc.ca/clinical_resource

3. Thrombosis Canada – https://thrombosiscanada.ca

4. Hypertension Canada Guidelines – https://hypertension.ca

5. CDC – https://www.cdc.gov/bloodpressure

HEART FAILURE AND ACUTE PULMONARY EDEMA — RURAL ER APPROACH

OVERVIEW

Acute decompensated heart failure with pulmonary edema is a life-threatening emergency.

It results from elevated left ventricular filling pressures leading to fluid accumulation in the lungs.

In rural ERs, rapid recognition, oxygenation, and initial pharmacological therapy are critical as access to advanced cardiac care may be limited.

CLINICAL PRESENTATION

1. Severe dyspnea, orthopnea, paroxysmal nocturnal dyspnea.
2. Cough with pink frothy sputum.
3. Hypoxemia, cyanosis.
4. Tachycardia, hypertension (early) or hypotension (late/shock).
5. Jugular venous distension, peripheral edema.

6.   Crackles/rales on auscultation, S3 gallop.

7.   Diaphoresis, anxiety, restlessness.

RED FLAGS

1.   Severe hypoxemia despite oxygen.

2.   Hypotension or cardiogenic shock.

3.   Altered mental status.

4.   Chest pain suggesting ACS.

5.   Ventricular arrhythmias or new AFib with rapid ventricular response.

DIFFERENTIAL DIAGNOSIS

1.   COPD/asthma exacerbation.

2.   Pneumonia or ARDS.

3.   Pulmonary embolism.

4.   Pneumothorax.

5.   Sepsis-related respiratory failure.

INVESTIGATIONS

1.   ECG: look for ischemia, arrhythmias.

2.   Labs: CBC, electrolytes, creatinine, troponin, BNP (if available).

3.   Chest X-ray: cardiomegaly, pulmonary edema.

4.   Point-of-care ultrasound: B-lines, pleural effusions, poor LV function.

5.   Bedside glucose and SpO_2 monitoring.

MANAGEMENT IN RURAL ER (WITH DRUG DOSAGES)

Immediate Stabilization:

1. Sit patient upright.
2. Oxygen 10–15 L/min by non-rebreather if hypoxemic; target $SpO_2 > 90\%$.
3. Non-invasive ventilation (CPAP 5–10 cmH_2O) if available; intubate if deteriorating.

Pharmacological Therapy:

1. Nitroglycerin: 0.4 mg SL q5min ×3 if SBP >100 mmHg. If persistent symptoms and SBP stable: IV infusion starting 5 mcg/min, titrate q5min by 5 mcg/min (max 200 mcg/min).
2. Furosemide: 20–40 mg IV bolus; if already on loop diuretic → give equal or higher IV dose than daily oral. Pediatrics: 1 mg/kg IV (max 6 mg/kg/day).
3. Morphine: 2–4 mg IV slow push q5–10min PRN for severe distress/anxiety (use cautiously due to risk of respiratory depression).

If Cardiogenic Shock:

1. Avoid aggressive nitrates/diuretics.
2. Consider inotropes: Dobutamine 2–20 mcg/kg/min IV infusion or Dopamine 5–20 mcg/kg/min IV infusion titrated to BP.
3. Norepinephrine 2–20 mcg/min IV infusion if hypotension refractory to fluids.

Additional:

1. Treat underlying triggers: ACS, arrhythmia, infection, uncontrolled hypertension.
2. Insert Foley catheter to monitor urine output.

WHEN TO CALL A SPECIALIST / TRANSFER

1. Severe pulmonary edema not improving after initial therapy.
2. Hypotension or cardiogenic shock.
3. ACS or arrhythmias requiring advanced interventions.
4. Recurrent decompensation.
5. Pediatric or pregnancy-related acute heart failure.
6. Early transfer arrangements should be made once stabilized.

DISPOSITION

1. Most patients require admission or transfer.
2. Safe discharge is rare; only if mild symptoms fully resolve and follow-up is ensured.
3. Admit locally if stable, monitoring available, and transfer not feasible immediately.
4. Transfer if unstable, requiring advanced cardiac support or invasive ventilation.

ADMISSION ORDERS (RURAL HOSPITAL)

1. Admit to monitored bed.
2. Oxygen as required.

3. Strict intake/output monitoring and daily weights.

4. IV furosemide as indicated.

5. Low-sodium diet, fluid restriction if appropriate.

6. Continue nitrates if symptomatic and BP stable.

7. Consider anticoagulation if immobile or AFib present.

8. Prepare for urgent transfer if deterioration occurs.

REFERENCES

1. Heart & Stroke Foundation of Canada – https://cpr. heartandstroke.ca

2. Emergency Care BC – https://emergencycarebc.ca/ clinical_resource

3. Canadian Cardiovascular Society Heart Failure Guidelines – https://ccs.ca

4. Thrombosis Canada – https://thrombosiscanada. ca

5. CDC – https://www.cdc.gov/heartdisease/heart_ failure.htm

CARDIAC ARREST & ACLS ALGORITHMS — RURAL ER APPROACH

OVERVIEW

Cardiac arrest is a sudden cessation of cardiac activity with loss of circulation and consciousness.

Immediate recognition and initiation of Advanced Cardiac Life Support (ACLS) are critical for survival.

In rural settings, limited personnel and delayed access to advanced interventions make adherence to simplified ACLS algorithms essential.

CLINICAL PRESENTATION

1. Unresponsive patient.
2. No normal breathing or only gasping.
3. No palpable pulse within 10 seconds.
4. ECG may show VF, pulseless VT, asystole, or PEA.

RED FLAGS

1. Prolonged downtime without CPR.

1. Severe hypothermia or toxin-related arrest (special considerations).

2. Pulseless electrical activity (PEA) — poor prognosis unless reversible cause treated.

3. Recurrent VF/VT despite shocks and medications.

DIFFERENTIAL DIAGNOSIS (REVERSIBLE CAUSES — HS & TS)

Hs:

1. Hypovolemia, Hypoxia, Hydrogen ion (acidosis), Hypo-/Hyperkalemia, Hypothermia.

Ts:

1. Tension pneumothorax, Tamponade (cardiac), Toxins, Thrombosis (MI/PE), Trauma.

INVESTIGATIONS

1. During cardiac arrest, investigations should not delay resuscitation.

2. Focus is on rapid ECG rhythm assessment, bedside glucose, and identifying reversible causes.

3. Post-ROSC (Return of Spontaneous Circulation): labs, CXR, ECG, troponins, and other investigations based

on suspected etiology.

MANAGEMENT IN RURAL ER (WITH DRUG DOSAGES)

Immediate actions:

1. Begin high-quality CPR immediately: 30:2 compressions to breaths (if no advanced airway), 100–120 compressions/min, depth 5–6 cm.
2. Attach monitor/defibrillator as soon as available.

Shockable rhythms (VF/pulseless VT):

1. Defibrillation: 200 J biphasic, repeat every 2 min as indicated.
2. Epinephrine: 1 mg IV/IO every 3–5 min during resuscitation.
3. Amiodarone: 300 mg IV/IO bolus after 2nd shock, may repeat 150 mg IV/IO once.

Non-shockable rhythms (PEA/Asystole):

1. Continue high-quality CPR.
2. Epinephrine: 1 mg IV/IO every 3–5 min.
3. Treat reversible causes (Hs and Ts).

Airway & Ventilation:

1. Bag-valve-mask with O_2; advanced airway if skilled provider available.
2. Once intubated: 1 breath every 6 sec (10 breaths/min), compressions continuous.

Post-ROSC Care:

1. Optimize oxygenation (SpO$_2$ 94–98%).

2. Maintain systolic BP ≥100 mmHg: fluids and vasopressors if needed.

3. Targeted temperature management (32–36°C) if available.

4. Early transfer to higher-level care for definitive treatment.

WHEN TO CALL A SPECIALIST / TRANSFER

1. After ROSC, all patients should be transferred to a higher-level facility for definitive management.

2. Consider early involvement of critical care transport teams.

3. Refractory arrhythmias, shock, or need for advanced post-arrest care warrant urgent transfer.

DISPOSITION

1. If ROSC achieved: stabilize and transfer.

2. If prolonged resuscitation without ROSC (>20–30 min) and no reversible cause identified → consider termination of efforts as per local policy.

3. Admit locally only if awaiting transfer and monitoring available.

ADMISSION ORDERS (RURAL HOSPITAL, POST-ROSC)

1. Admit to monitored/ICU bed if available.

2. Continuous ECG, SpO_2, BP monitoring.

3. Oxygen to maintain SpO_2 94–98%.

4. IV fluids as needed to maintain BP.

5. Vasopressors: norepinephrine infusion 2–20 mcg/min IV titrated.

6. Targeted temperature management if feasible.

7. Arrange urgent transfer.

REFERENCE

1. Heart & Stroke Foundation of Canada — Advanced Cardiac Life Support (ACLS) Guidelines: https://cpr.heartandstroke.ca

SECTION III –
RESPIRATORY EMERGENCIES

ACUTE ASTHMA EXACERBATION — RURAL ER APPROACH

OVERVIEW

Acute asthma exacerbations are a common presentation to rural emergency departments. They range from mild to life-threatening. Limited resources in rural settings necessitate early recognition, prompt treatment, and clear transfer criteria. The goals are rapid reversal of airflow obstruction, oxygenation, and prevention of respiratory failure.

CLINICAL PRESENTATION

1. Dyspnea, wheezing, cough, chest tightness.
2. Increased respiratory rate and accessory muscle use.
3. Hypoxemia (low SpO_2), tachycardia.
4. Severe cases: silent chest, altered mental status, cyanosis, exhaustion.
5. Pediatric differences: may present with retractions, inability to feed, agitation or drowsiness.

RED FLAGS

1. Silent chest or minimal air movement.
2. SpO_2 < 90% despite oxygen therapy.
3. Severe tachypnea, inability to speak in full sentences.
4. Altered mental status, exhaustion, impending respiratory arrest.
5. Hypotension or pulsus paradoxus.

DIFFERENTIAL DIAGNOSIS

1. COPD exacerbation.
2. Pneumonia.
3. Upper airway obstruction (foreign body, anaphylaxis).
4. Pulmonary embolism.
5. Heart failure with pulmonary edema.

INVESTIGATIONS

1. Primarily a clinical diagnosis — do not delay treatment.
2. Bedside: SpO_2, vitals, peak expiratory flow (if able).
3. ECG: to exclude arrhythmia or ACS in adults.
4. CXR if alternate diagnosis suspected.
5. Labs (if available): CBC, electrolytes, VBG/ABG in severe cases.

MANAGEMENT IN RURAL ER (WITH DRUG DOSAGES)

Immediate management:

1. Oxygen: administer to maintain $SpO_2 \geq 92\%$ in adults, $\geq 94\%$ in children.

Bronchodilators:

1. Salbutamol (albuterol): 2.5–5 mg via nebulizer q20min for 3 doses, then 2.5–10 mg q1–4h PRN;

MDI with spacer 4–8 puffs q20min ×3, then q1–4h PRN. Pediatrics: 0.15 mg/kg/dose (min 2.5 mg, max 5 mg) q20min ×3.

1. Ipratropium bromide: 0.5 mg nebulized q20min ×3, then q2–4h PRN. Pediatrics: 250 mcg/dose nebulized q20min ×3.

Corticosteroids:

1. Prednisone: Adults 40–60 mg PO daily ×5 days.
2. Pediatrics: Prednisone/Prednisolone 1–2 mg/kg PO daily (max 50 mg).
3. If unable to take PO: Methylprednisolone 125 mg IV (adults) or 1–2 mg/kg IV (pediatrics, max 60 mg).

Adjuncts:

1. Magnesium sulfate: 2 g IV over 20 min (adults); Pediatrics: 25–75 mg/kg IV over 20 min (max 2 g) for severe cases.

2. Epinephrine (if impending respiratory failure, or concern for anaphylaxis): 0.3–0.5 mg IM (1:1000) q20min ×3; Pediatrics: 0.01 mg/kg IM (max 0.3 mg).

If impending arrest:

1. Prepare for intubation (Ketamine 1–2 mg/kg IV, Rocuronium 1.2 mg/kg IV). Intubation should be last resort due to risk of complications.

WHEN TO CALL A SPECIALIST / TRANSFER

1. Severe or life-threatening exacerbation.
2. Failure to improve after initial therapy.
3. Need for IV magnesium or epinephrine.
4. Impending respiratory failure or need for intubation.
5. Pediatric severe exacerbation not responding to treatment.
6. Early transfer arrangements recommended in all severe cases.

DISPOSITION

1. Discharge: only if symptoms fully resolve, $SpO_2 \geq 94\%$ on room air, PEFR $\geq 70\%$ predicted, and patient has access to follow-up and inhalers.
2. Admit locally: if moderate symptoms persist and monitoring available.
3. Transfer: all patients with severe/life-threatening features or requiring advanced support.

ADMISSION ORDERS (RURAL HOSPITAL)

1. Admit to monitored bed.

2. Salbutamol via nebulizer or MDI q1–4h.

3. Ipratropium q4–6h for first 24h if severe.

4. Prednisone/Prednisolone as above.

5. Oxygen to maintain SpO_2 target.

6. Continuous monitoring if severe.

7. Prepare for transfer if deteriorating.

REFERENCES

1. Emergency Care BC – https://emergencycarebc.ca/clinical_resource

2. Canadian Paediatric Society – https://cps.ca

3. Heart & Stroke Foundation of Canada – https://cpr.heartandstroke.ca

4. CDC Asthma – https://www.cdc.gov/asthma

5. WHO Emergency Care Guidance – https://www.who.int

COPD EXACERBATION — RURAL ER APPROACH

OVERVIEW

Acute exacerbations of chronic obstructive pulmonary disease (COPD) are common presentations in the rural ER.

They are often triggered by infection, environmental exposure, or nonadherence to medications. Exacerbations range from mild to life-threatening.

Rural clinicians must focus on early oxygenation, bronchodilation, corticosteroids, and antibiotics when indicated, while preparing for transfer in severe cases.

CLINICAL PRESENTATION

1. Increased dyspnea, cough, sputum volume, or purulence.
2. Hypoxemia, tachypnea, wheezing, prolonged expiration.
3. Use of accessory muscles, tripod positioning.
4. Severe: confusion, cyanosis, inability to speak in

full sentences, impending respiratory failure.

5. History of smoking, occupational exposures, recurrent exacerbations.

RED FLAGS

1. $SpO_2 < 90\%$ despite oxygen.
2. Altered mental status, confusion.
3. Severe tachypnea, accessory muscle fatigue.
4. Silent chest or absent breath sounds.
5. Hypotension or arrhythmias.
6. Suspicion of pneumothorax or pneumonia complicating COPD.

DIFFERENTIAL DIAGNOSIS

1. Asthma exacerbation.
2. Pneumonia.
3. Pulmonary embolism.
4. Heart failure with pulmonary edema.
5. Upper airway obstruction.

INVESTIGATIONS

1. Bedside: SpO_2, vitals.
2. ECG: assess for arrhythmia, ischemia.
3. CXR: pneumonia, pneumothorax, CHF.
4. Labs: CBC, electrolytes, creatinine, ABG/VBG ($PaCO_2$ retention, acidosis).
5. Sputum culture if infectious cause suspected.

MANAGEMENT IN RURAL ER (WITH DRUG DOSAGES)

Oxygen:

1. Target SpO_2 88–92% (avoid over-oxygenation in CO_2 retainers).
2. Nasal cannula or Venturi mask preferred; escalate to NRB mask or NIV if severe.

Bronchodilators:

1. Salbutamol: 2.5 mg nebulized q20min ×3, then 2.5–10 mg q1–4h PRN; MDI 4–8 puffs q20min ×3, then q1–4h PRN.
2. Ipratropium: 0.5 mg nebulized q20min ×3, then q2–6h. MDI: 4–8 puffs q20min ×3, then q2–4h.

Corticosteroids:

1. Prednisone 40 mg PO daily ×5 days (adults).
2. If unable to take PO: Methylprednisolone 125 mg IV once, then 40 mg IV q12h.

Antibiotics (if increased sputum purulence, volume, or need for ventilation):

1. Amoxicillin-clavulanate 875 mg PO BID ×5–7 days.
2. Doxycycline 100 mg PO BID ×5–7 days.
3. Azithromycin 500 mg PO day 1, then 250 mg PO daily ×4 days.

Adjuncts:

1. Magnesium sulfate: 2 g IV over 20 min for severe bronchospasm.
2. Consider furosemide 20–40 mg IV if overlapping CHF suspected.

Impending Respiratory Failure:
1. Non-invasive ventilation (BiPAP) if available.
2. Prepare for intubation (Ketamine 1–2 mg/kg IV, Rocuronium 1.2 mg/kg IV).

WHEN TO CALL A SPECIALIST / TRANSFER

1. Severe COPD exacerbation requiring NIV or intubation.
2. Failure to respond to initial therapy.
3. Recurrent exacerbations with poor baseline function.
4. Suspected pneumothorax, pneumonia, or PE complicating COPD.
5. Pediatric transfer not applicable; adult transfer if unstable or requiring ICU-level care.

DISPOSITION

1. Discharge: if mild, improved after treatment, SpO_2 stable 90–92% on room air or home O_2, reliable follow-up.
2. Admit locally: if persistent hypoxemia, need for frequent nebulizers, poor social support.
3. Transfer: if requiring NIV, intubation, or

complicated by pneumonia, CHF, or shock.

ADMISSION ORDERS (RURAL HOSPITAL)

1. Oxygen to maintain SpO_2 88–92%.
2. Salbutamol and Ipratropium nebulizers q4–6h, plus PRN.
3. Prednisone 40 mg PO daily (or IV methylprednisolone if unable to take PO).
4. Empiric antibiotics if indicated.
5. Monitor for CO_2 retention, repeat ABG if available.
6. Consider DVT prophylaxis if immobile.
7. Prepare for transfer if deterioration occurs.

REFERENCES

1. Emergency Care BC – https://emergencycarebc.ca/clinical_resource
2. Canadian Thoracic Society COPD Guidelines (open summaries) – https://cts-sct.ca
3. CDC COPD – https://www.cdc.gov/copd
4. WHO Emergency Care Guidance – https://www.who.int

PNEUMONIA IN ADULTS & CHILDREN (COMMUNITY-ACQUIRED PNEUMONIA, CAP) — RURAL ER APPROACH

OVERVIEW

Community-acquired pneumonia (CAP) is a leading cause of morbidity and mortality worldwide.

In rural ERs, challenges include limited diagnostic tools, resource constraints, and transfer delays.

Management requires early recognition, empiric antibiotics, and supportive care while identifying those who need admission or transfer.

CLINICAL PRESENTATION

Adults:
1. Cough, fever, chills, dyspnea, pleuritic chest pain.
2. Tachypnea, tachycardia, hypoxemia.
3. Crackles, bronchial breath sounds, dullness to

percussion.

Children:

1. Fever, cough, tachypnea (age-specific RR thresholds: >60/min <2mo, >50/min 2–12mo, >40/min 1–5yr).
2. Chest indrawing, grunting, nasal flaring, poor feeding, lethargy.
3. Crackles, decreased air entry, wheeze (sometimes).

RED FLAGS

1. SpO_2 < 90% on room air.
2. Severe respiratory distress, exhaustion.
3. Altered mental status, lethargy, apnea in infants.
4. Hypotension, septic shock.
5. Inability to maintain oral intake or dehydration.
6. Neonates and infants <2 months — high risk of rapid deterioration.

DIFFERENTIAL DIAGNOSIS

1. Viral bronchitis or bronchiolitis.
2. Asthma/COPD exacerbation.
3. Pulmonary embolism.
4. Heart failure with pulmonary edema.
5. TB (subacute course).

INVESTIGATIONS

1. Primarily a clinical diagnosis in rural settings.

2. Bedside: vitals, SpO_2.

3. CXR if available, but do not delay treatment.

4. Labs: CBC, electrolytes, blood culture if severe.

5. Consider viral testing during outbreaks (influenza, RSV, COVID).

MANAGEMENT IN RURAL ER (WITH DRUG DOSAGES)

Supportive:

1. Oxygen to maintain $SpO_2 \geq 92\%$ adults, $\geq 94\%$ children.

2. IV fluids if dehydrated: Adults 500–1000 mL NS bolus; Pediatrics 20 mL/kg bolus if shock.

Empiric Antibiotics (Adults):

1. Outpatient: Amoxicillin 1 g PO TID ×5–7 days OR Doxycycline 100 mg PO BID ×5–7 days.

2. Inpatient (moderate): Ceftriaxone 1–2 g IV daily + Azithromycin 500 mg PO/IV daily.

3. Severe: Ceftriaxone 2 g IV daily + Azithromycin 500 mg IV daily, consider Vancomycin if MRSA risk.

Empiric Antibiotics (Children):

1. Outpatient: Amoxicillin 80–90 mg/kg/day PO ÷2–3 doses (max 3 g/day).

2. Inpatient (moderate): Ampicillin 200 mg/kg/day IV ÷4 doses OR Ceftriaxone 50 mg/kg IV daily (max 2 g).

3. Severe: Ceftriaxone 50 mg/kg IV daily (max 2 g) +

Azithromycin 10 mg/kg PO/IV daily (max 500 mg).

4. Add Vancomycin 15 mg/kg IV q6h (max 2 g/day) if MRSA suspected.

Adjuncts:

1. Antipyretics: Acetaminophen 650–1000 mg PO/IV q6h (max 4 g/day adults); Pediatrics 15 mg/kg PO/IV q6h (max 75 mg/kg/day).

2. Ibuprofen: Adults 400 mg PO q6–8h (max 2400 mg/day); Pediatrics 10 mg/kg PO q6–8h (max 40 mg/kg/day).

3. Nebulized bronchodilators if bronchospasm present.

If impending respiratory failure:

1. Prepare for advanced airway (Ketamine 1–2 mg/kg IV, Rocuronium 1.2 mg/kg IV if intubation required).

WHEN TO CALL A SPECIALIST / TRANSFER

1. Severe pneumonia with hypoxemia, shock, or altered mental status.

2. Pediatric patients with moderate–severe pneumonia, especially <2 months old.

3. Failure to respond to initial therapy.

4. Complications: empyema, effusion, abscess.

5. Need for mechanical ventilation or ICU-level care.

DISPOSITION

1. Discharge: only if mild, stable, SpO_2 normal on room

air, and reliable follow-up.

2. Admit locally: if moderate, requiring IV antibiotics or oxygen, but stable.

3. Transfer: if severe, requiring advanced respiratory or hemodynamic support.

ADMISSION ORDERS (RURAL HOSPITAL)

1. Admit to monitored bed.

2. Oxygen to maintain SpO_2.

3. IV antibiotics as above.

4. IV fluids for hydration.

5. Antipyretics for fever.

6. Continuous monitoring if severe.

7. Prepare for urgent transfer if deterioration occurs.

REFERENCES

1. Emergency Care BC – https://emergencycarebc.ca/clinical_resource

2. Canadian Paediatric Society – https://cps.ca

3. CDC Pneumonia – https://www.cdc.gov/pneumonia

4. WHO Pneumonia Care Guidance – https://www.who.int

ANAPHYLAXIS (RECOGNITION & EPINEPHRINE DOSING) — RURAL ER APPROACH

OVERVIEW

Anaphylaxis is a severe, life-threatening systemic hypersensitivity reaction that requires immediate recognition and treatment.

In rural ERs, rapid administration of intramuscular epinephrine is the cornerstone of management. Delays in treatment are associated with mortality.

Supportive measures and preparation for transfer are critical.

CLINICAL PRESENTATION

1. Sudden onset (minutes to hours) after exposure to allergen (food, insect sting, medication).
2. Skin: urticaria, flushing, angioedema.
3. Respiratory: stridor, wheeze, dyspnea, throat

tightness.

4. Cardiovascular: hypotension, dizziness, syncope, shock.

5. GI: nausea, vomiting, abdominal pain, diarrhea.

6. Severe: airway obstruction, cardiovascular collapse, cardiac arrest.

RED FLAGS

1. Hypotension or shock.

2. Stridor, wheezing, or airway compromise.

3. Rapid progression of symptoms.

4. History of prior anaphylaxis.

5. Poor response to initial epinephrine dose.

DIFFERENTIAL DIAGNOSIS

1. Vasovagal syncope.

2. Asthma attack.

3. Sepsis.

4. Angioedema (non-allergic, e.g., ACE inhibitor induced).

5. Panic attack.

INVESTIGATIONS

1. Clinical diagnosis — investigations should not delay treatment.

2. SpO_2, ECG, BP, bedside glucose if altered LOC.

3. Labs (after stabilization): CBC, electrolytes, serum

tryptase (if available).

MANAGEMENT IN RURAL ER (WITH DRUG DOSAGES)

First-line treatment:

1. Epinephrine (1:1000, 1 mg/mL): Adults: 0.3–0.5 mg IM in mid-thigh, q5–15min PRN. Pediatrics: 0.01 mg/kg IM (max 0.3 mg) q5–15min PRN.
2. Give immediately at first signs of anaphylaxis — do not delay.

Airway & Breathing:

1. Oxygen 10–15 L/min by non-rebreather mask.
2. Prepare for intubation if airway swelling progresses (Ketamine 1–2 mg/kg IV, Rocuronium 1.2 mg/kg IV).

Circulation:

1. Place patient supine with legs elevated unless respiratory distress.
2. IV fluids: Normal saline bolus 1–2 L in adults; Pediatrics: 20 mL/kg bolus, repeat as needed.

Adjuncts (AFTER epinephrine):

1. Antihistamines: Diphenhydramine 25–50 mg IV/IM (Pediatrics: 1 mg/kg IV/IM, max 50 mg).
2. Ranitidine (if available): 50 mg IV diluted in 5% dextrose over 5 min (less common now).
3. Corticosteroids: Methylprednisolone 125 mg IV or

Prednisone 40–60 mg PO; Pediatrics: Prednisone 1–2 mg/kg PO (max 50 mg).

Bronchospasm not relieved by epinephrine:
1. Salbutamol 2.5–5 mg nebulized q20min PRN (Pediatrics: 0.15 mg/kg nebulized, min 2.5 mg, max 5 mg).

Refractory anaphylaxis:
1. Epinephrine infusion: 1 mg epinephrine in 1000 mL NS = 1 mcg/mL; start at 1 mcg/min, titrate 1–10 mcg/min to maintain BP.
2. Vasopressors (if available): Norepinephrine 2–20 mcg/min IV infusion if persistent shock.

WHEN TO CALL A SPECIALIST / TRANSFER

1. All anaphylaxis patients require transfer or observation for ≥4–6 hours (biphasic reactions possible).
2. Severe cases requiring >2 doses epinephrine, airway management, or IV vasopressors should be transferred to ICU-level care.
3. Pediatric patients with airway compromise or hypotension require urgent transfer.

DISPOSITION

1. Discharge: Only after full resolution, observation ≥4–6 hours, access to follow-up, and prescription of epinephrine auto-injector.
2. Admit locally: If recurrent symptoms or comorbidities.

3. Transfer: If severe, required intubation, or persistent hypotension/shock.

ADMISSION ORDERS (RURAL HOSPITAL)

1. Admit to monitored bed.
2. Continuous SpO_2, ECG, BP monitoring.
3. Oxygen as needed.
4. IV access and fluids as required.
5. Corticosteroids PO/IV for prevention of biphasic reaction.
6. Epinephrine auto-injector prescribed before discharge.
7. Arrange follow-up with allergy specialist if available.

REFERENCES

1. Canadian Paediatric Society – https://cps.ca
2. Emergency Care BC – https://emergencycarebc.ca/clinical_resource
3. CDC Anaphylaxis Guidance – https://www.cdc.gov
4. World Allergy Organization – https://www.worldallergy.org
5. WHO Emergency Care Guidelines – https://www.who.int

UPPER AIRWAY EMERGENCIES (EPIGLOTTITIS, FOREIGN BODY, ANGIOEDEMA) — RURAL ER APPROACH

OVERVIEW

Upper airway emergencies such as epiglottitis, foreign body aspiration, and angioedema are life-threatening conditions requiring rapid recognition and management. In rural ERs, limited resources and delayed access to surgical airway specialists make early airway protection and transfer planning critical.

CLINICAL PRESENTATION

Epiglottitis:
1. Sudden onset sore throat, dysphagia, drooling, muffled "hot potato" voice.
2. Stridor, respiratory distress, sitting forward (tripod position).
3. Children: appear toxic, anxious, drooling.

Foreign Body Aspiration:

1. Sudden choking, cough, stridor, unilateral wheeze, decreased breath sounds.

2. In severe cases: cyanosis, inability to speak or cough.

Angioedema:

1. Swelling of lips, tongue, face, airway.

2. May progress rapidly to airway obstruction.

3. Often associated with allergic reactions, ACE inhibitors, or hereditary angioedema.

RED FLAGS

1. Stridor or severe respiratory distress.

2. Inability to swallow, drooling.

3. Cyanosis, hypoxemia.

4. Altered mental status, exhaustion.

5. Rapid progression of swelling (angioedema).

DIFFERENTIAL DIAGNOSIS

1. Asthma, COPD exacerbation.

2. Croup.

3. Anaphylaxis without airway edema.

4. Peritonsillar abscess.

5. Retropharyngeal abscess.

INVESTIGATIONS

1. Clinical diagnosis — do NOT delay airway management.

2. Avoid agitating children with suspected epiglottitis (no throat exam with tongue depressor).
3. Bedside: SpO_2, vitals.
4. Lateral neck X-ray may show "thumb sign" in epiglottitis, but only if stable.
5. CXR if foreign body aspiration suspected and patient stable.

MANAGEMENT IN RURAL ER (WITH DRUG DOSAGES)

General Principles:
1. Prepare for difficult airway; early call for anesthesia/ ENT if available.
2. Do not agitate patient; keep sitting upright if tolerated.
3. If severe obstruction → prepare for surgical airway (needle cricothyrotomy if unable to ventilate/intubate).

Epiglottitis:
1. Oxygen as tolerated.
2. Ceftriaxone 2 g IV daily (adults) or 50 mg/kg IV daily (pediatrics, max 2 g).
3. Dexamethasone 10 mg IV (pediatrics: 0.6 mg/kg IV, max 10 mg).

Foreign Body Aspiration:
1. Complete obstruction: Heimlich maneuver (adults/ children >1 yr) or 5 back blows + 5 chest thrusts (infants <1 yr).

2. Partial obstruction: keep patient calm, prepare for rigid bronchoscopy if available.

3. If patient collapses/unresponsive: start CPR, attempt visualization and removal with Magill forceps if object visible.

Angioedema:

1. Airway: prepare for intubation or cricothyrotomy if needed.

2. Epinephrine IM (1:1000, 1 mg/mL): Adults 0.3–0.5 mg IM q5–15min; Pediatrics 0.01 mg/kg IM (max 0.3 mg).

3. Diphenhydramine 25–50 mg IV/IM (pediatrics: 1 mg/kg, max 50 mg).

4. Methylprednisolone 125 mg IV (pediatrics: 1–2 mg/kg IV, max 60 mg).

5. Tranexamic Acid (TXA): 1 g IV over 10 min for ACE inhibitor angioedema (limited evidence but used in practice).

6. If hereditary angioedema: C1 esterase inhibitor concentrate 20 units/kg IV (if available).

WHEN TO CALL A SPECIALIST / TRANSFER

1. All cases with threatened or established airway compromise.

2. Pediatric epiglottitis (high risk of sudden deterioration).

3. Foreign body not retrievable locally.

4. Angioedema requiring repeated epinephrine or airway intervention.

5. Arrange early transfer to facility with ENT/

anesthesia backup.

DISPOSITION

1. Discharge: only if mild angioedema without airway involvement and good follow-up.
2. Admit locally: if moderate, stable after treatment, and airway secure.
3. Transfer: most epiglottitis, severe angioedema, and foreign body aspiration cases require higher-level care.

ADMISSION ORDERS (RURAL HOSPITAL)

1. Admit to monitored bed.
2. Oxygen as needed.
3. Airway equipment and emergency drugs at bedside.
4. IV antibiotics for epiglottitis, steroids, antihistamines for angioedema.
5. Prepare for rapid deterioration and urgent transfer if required.

REFERENCES

1. Emergency Care BC – https://emergencycarebc.ca/clinical_resource
2. Canadian Paediatric Society – https://cps.ca
3. CDC – https://www.cdc.gov
4. WHO Emergency Care Guidance – https://www.who.int

RESPIRATORY DISTRESS IN INFANTS (BRONCHIOLITIS, CROUP) — RURAL ER APPROACH

OVERVIEW

Respiratory distress in infants is a frequent cause of emergency visits.

Bronchiolitis and viral croup are two of the most common conditions.

Rural ER providers must rapidly identify severity, provide supportive care, and escalate management when needed.

Most cases are viral, self-limited, but severe presentations may require transfer.

CLINICAL PRESENTATION

Bronchiolitis (common in infants <2 years, usually RSV):
1. Rhinorrhea, cough, fever, poor feeding.
2. Tachypnea, wheezing, crackles, nasal flaring,

retractions.

3. Apnea in very young infants.

Croup (usually ages 6 months – 3 years):

1. Barking cough, inspiratory stridor, hoarseness.

2. Symptoms worse at night.

3. Severe: stridor at rest, retractions, hypoxemia, agitation or lethargy.

RED FLAGS

1. $SpO_2 < 90\%$ on room air.

2. Severe chest retractions, nasal flaring, grunting.

3. Lethargy, poor feeding, dehydration.

4. Apnea or cyanosis.

5. Stridor at rest (croup).

6. Exhaustion or altered LOC.

DIFFERENTIAL DIAGNOSIS

1. Asthma/reactive airway disease.

2. Foreign body aspiration.

3. Pneumonia.

4. Congenital heart disease.

5. Upper airway obstruction (e.g., epiglottitis).

INVESTIGATIONS

1. Primarily clinical diagnosis.

2. Bedside: SpO_2, vitals.

3. CXR if severe distress or uncertain diagnosis.

4. Labs rarely indicated unless sepsis suspected.

5. Viral swabs may confirm diagnosis but not required for management.

MANAGEMENT IN RURAL ER (WITH DRUG DOSAGES)

Bronchiolitis:

1. Supportive care is mainstay.

2. Oxygen if SpO_2 < 90%.

3. Nasal suctioning for secretions.

4. Hydration: IV/NG fluids if unable to feed.

5. Nebulized epinephrine or bronchodilators are generally not effective, but may trial if severe and reassess.

Croup:

1. Mild (no stridor at rest): Dexamethasone 0.15–0.6 mg/kg PO/IM/IV (max 16 mg).

2. Moderate/severe (stridor at rest, retractions):

   • Dexamethasone 0.6 mg/kg PO/IM/IV (max 16 mg).

   • Nebulized epinephrine: 0.5 mL of 2.25% solution in 2.5 mL NS via nebulizer; may repeat q20min ×3.

If impending respiratory failure (bronchiolitis or croup):

1. Prepare for advanced airway (Ketamine 1–2 mg/kg IV, Rocuronium 1.2 mg/kg IV if intubation unavoidable).

2. Call for transfer to pediatric-capable facility.

Adjuncts:

1. Antipyretics: Acetaminophen 15 mg/kg PO/PR/IV q6h PRN (max 75 mg/kg/day).

2. Ibuprofen 10 mg/kg PO q6–8h PRN (max 40 mg/kg/day; only if >6 months old).

WHEN TO CALL A SPECIALIST / TRANSFER

1. Infants with severe distress, apnea, hypoxemia, or dehydration.

2. Failure to improve with initial therapy.

3. Need for repeated nebulized epinephrine.

4. Infants <2 months old with suspected bronchiolitis.

5. Consider early transfer if resources limited.

DISPOSITION

1. Discharge: if feeding well, no hypoxemia, mild symptoms, reliable caregivers.

2. Admit locally: if moderate distress, need for O_2, IV fluids, or close monitoring.

3. Transfer: if severe distress, apnea, or requiring repeated nebulized epinephrine or advanced airway support.

ADMISSION ORDERS (RURAL HOSPITAL)

1. Oxygen to maintain $SpO_2 > 90\%$.

2. IV/NG fluids for hydration.

3. Dexamethasone for croup.

4. Nebulized epinephrine for severe croup.

5. Antipyretics for fever.

6. Continuous monitoring in severe cases.

7. Arrange transfer if unstable or worsening.

REFERENCES

1. Canadian Paediatric Society – https://cps.ca

2. Emergency Care BC – https://emergencycarebc.ca/clinical_resource

3. CDC Bronchiolitis – https://www.cdc.gov

4. WHO Childhood Respiratory Infections – https://www.who.int

SECTION IV –
NEUROLOGICAL EMERGENCIES

ACUTE STROKE (RECOGNITION, TPA/ TRANSFER CRITERIA) — RURAL ER APPROACH

OVERVIEW

Stroke is a leading cause of morbidity and mortality. Early recognition and timely reperfusion therapy significantly improve outcomes. In rural ERs, challenges include limited imaging availability and transfer delays. Focus is on rapid recognition, stabilization, and immediate consultation with a stroke center for potential thrombolysis or thrombectomy.

CLINICAL PRESENTATION

1. Sudden onset focal neurological deficit: weakness, numbness, speech difficulty, vision loss.
2. Hemiparesis, facial droop, dysarthria, aphasia.
3. Ataxia, vertigo, imbalance.
4. Severe headache (suggests hemorrhagic stroke).
5. Altered level of consciousness in severe cases.

RED FLAGS

1. Airway compromise or decreased LOC.

2. Rapid progression of neurological deficit.

3. Severe hypertension (SBP > 220 mmHg or DBP > 120 mmHg).

4. Seizures at onset.

5. Signs of raised intracranial pressure (bradycardia, irregular breathing, hypertension).

DIFFERENTIAL DIAGNOSIS

1. Hypoglycemia (always check glucose).

2. Seizure with Todd's paralysis.

3. Migraine with aura.

4. CNS infection (meningitis/encephalitis).

5. Brain tumor or abscess.

INVESTIGATIONS

1. Bedside glucose (rule out hypoglycemia).

2. Non-contrast CT head (to rule out hemorrhage) — essential before thrombolysis.

3. ECG, CBC, electrolytes, creatinine, INR/PTT if available.

4. Oxygen saturation, BP monitoring.

5. If CT not available in rural ER — initiate transfer immediately after stabilization.

MANAGEMENT IN RURAL ER (WITH DRUG DOSAGES)

Stabilization:

1. Oxygen if SpO_2 < 94%.
2. Maintain BP unless >220/120 mmHg (ischemic stroke) or >185/110 mmHg if candidate for tPA.
3. IV labetalol 10–20 mg IV over 1–2 min, may repeat q10min (max 300 mg) OR infusion 2 mg/min for BP lowering.
4. IV hydralazine 10 mg IV q20min PRN as alternative.

Thrombolysis (tPA, Alteplase):

1. Indicated for ischemic stroke if onset <4.5 hours, no contraindications, and confirmed on CT.
2. Dose: 0.9 mg/kg IV (max 90 mg): 10% IV bolus over 1 min, remainder infused over 60 min.
3. Contraindications: hemorrhage on CT, recent surgery, active bleeding, INR >1.7, platelets <100, uncontrolled BP >185/110.

Antiplatelet (if not candidate for tPA and hemorrhage excluded):

1. Aspirin 160–325 mg PO chewed once, then 81 mg daily.

Transfer Criteria:

1. All suspected stroke patients should be transferred to

a stroke center.

2. tPA-eligible: initiate treatment (if possible) before transfer.

3. Suspected large vessel occlusion (LVO): transfer for thrombectomy if within 6–24h window.

WHEN TO CALL A SPECIALIST / TRANSFER

1. All suspected acute stroke patients require neurology consultation.

2. Immediately contact regional stroke center via telestroke (if available).

3. Transfer urgently if CT or thrombolysis not available locally.

4. Pediatric stroke requires specialized center transfer.

DISPOSITION

1. Transfer most acute stroke patients to stroke-capable center.

2. Admit locally only if minor stroke/TIA with complete resolution and access to rapid follow-up.

3. All tPA-treated patients require ICU/step-down monitoring after transfer.

ADMISSION ORDERS (RURAL HOSPITAL, IF AWAITING TRANSFER)

1. Admit to monitored bed.

2. NPO until swallow assessment completed.

3. Oxygen to maintain $SpO_2 \geq 94\%$.

4. Neuro checks q1h.

5. Maintain BP as per ischemic vs hemorrhagic criteria.

6. IV fluids: NS 75–100 mL/hr (avoid dextrose solutions).

7. Aspirin 160 mg PO/PR if not candidate for tPA and hemorrhage excluded.

REFERENCES

1. Heart & Stroke Foundation of Canada – Stroke Best Practice Guidelines: https://www.strokebestpractices. ca

2. Emergency Care BC – https://emergencycarebc.ca/ clinical_resource

3. CDC Stroke – https://www.cdc.gov/stroke

4. WHO Stroke Guidance – https://www.who.int

SEIZURES AND STATUS EPILEPTICUS — RURAL ER APPROACH

OVERVIEW

Seizures are common neurological emergencies. Status epilepticus (SE) is defined as a seizure lasting >5 minutes or recurrent seizures without recovery of consciousness between episodes. SE is life-threatening, requiring rapid intervention to prevent hypoxia, brain injury, and death. Rural ERs must prioritize airway, rapid pharmacologic therapy, and early transfer if refractory.

CLINICAL PRESENTATION

1. Generalized tonic–clonic movements, loss of consciousness.
2. Focal seizures: twitching, automatisms, altered awareness.
3. Non-convulsive SE: prolonged confusion, subtle twitching, coma.
4. Associated: tongue biting, incontinence, post-ictal drowsiness.

RED FLAGS

1. Seizure lasting >5 minutes (status epilepticus).
2. Recurrent seizures without regaining consciousness.
3. Hypoxemia, cyanosis.
4. Hypotension, arrhythmias.
5. Associated trauma or suspected CNS infection.

DIFFERENTIAL DIAGNOSIS

1. Syncope.
2. Hypoglycemia.
3. Psychogenic non-epileptic seizures.
4. Stroke, TIA.
5. Electrolyte disturbance (Na, Ca, Mg).

INVESTIGATIONS

1. Bedside glucose (treat hypoglycemia if present).
2. CBC, electrolytes, calcium, magnesium, creatinine.
3. Toxicology screen if suspected ingestion.
4. Head CT if first seizure, trauma, or focal deficit.
5. ECG, SpO_2 monitoring.

MANAGEMENT IN RURAL ER (WITH DRUG DOSAGES)

Immediate stabilization:

1. Airway: protect, position, suction secretions, give O_2.
2. If unable to protect airway: prepare for intubation

(Ketamine 1–2 mg/kg IV, Rocuronium 1.2 mg/kg IV).

First-line (benzodiazepines):

1. Lorazepam 0.1 mg/kg IV (max 4 mg/dose), may repeat in 5–10 min.
2. Diazepam 0.2 mg/kg IV (max 10 mg/dose), may repeat q10–15min (max 30 mg).
3. Midazolam 0.2 mg/kg IM/IN (max 10 mg) if no IV access.

Second-line (antiepileptics):

1. Phenytoin 20 mg/kg IV (max 1500 mg) at ≤50 mg/min; may give additional 5–10 mg/kg if needed.
2. Fosphenytoin 20 mg PE/kg IV at ≤1500 mg PE/min.
3. Valproate 20–40 mg/kg IV over 10 min (max 3000 mg).
4. Levetiracetam 60 mg/kg IV over 15 min (max 4500 mg).

Refractory SE (persistent after benzo + 2nd line):

1. Midazolam infusion: 0.05–2 mg/kg/hr.
2. Propofol infusion: 2–5 mg/kg loading, then 2–10 mg/kg/hr.
3. Phenobarbital 15–20 mg/kg IV (max 1000 mg).

Correct underlying causes:

1. Hypoglycemia: Dextrose 25 g IV (50 mL D50W); Pediatrics: D10W 5 mL/kg IV.
2. Thiamine 100 mg IV before glucose in alcoholics/

malnourished.

3. Electrolyte replacement (Na, Ca, Mg) as indicated.

WHEN TO CALL A SPECIALIST / TRANSFER

1. All patients with status epilepticus not rapidly controlled.

2. Suspected CNS infection, trauma, stroke.

3. Pediatric SE requiring escalation of care.

4. Refractory seizures requiring continuous infusion and ICU support.

5. Early neurology/critical care consultation recommended.

DISPOSITION

1. Admit locally: only if first seizure, stable, resolved, normal neuro exam, and follow-up available.

2. Transfer: all SE patients, refractory seizures, or requiring advanced airway/ventilation.

3. Discharge: possible if single seizure with known epilepsy, full recovery, normal exam, and reliable follow-up.

ADMISSION ORDERS (RURAL HOSPITAL)

1. Admit to monitored bed.

2. Seizure precautions, continuous ECG and SpO_2.

3. IV access, maintain airway and O_2.

4. Antiepileptic maintenance: phenytoin, valproate, or levetiracetam.

5. Thiamine and glucose if indicated.

6. Prepare for transfer if recurrent seizures or refractory SE.

REFERENCES

1. Emergency Care BC – https://emergencycarebc.ca/clinical_resource

2. Canadian Paediatric Society – https://cps.ca

3. CDC Seizure Guidance – https://www.cdc.gov/epilepsy

4. WHO Emergency Care Guidelines – https://www.who.int

HEAD INJURY (ADULT & PEDIATRIC CONCUSSION/TRAUMA) — RURAL ER APPROACH

OVERVIEW

Head injuries range from concussion (mild traumatic brain injury, mTBI) to severe traumatic brain injury (TBI). In rural ERs, priorities are early recognition of red flags, prevention of secondary brain injury (avoid hypotension, hypoxemia), judicious imaging, and deciding between observation, local admission, or urgent transfer. Use open-access, validated decision rules and guidelines for both adults and children.

CLINICAL PRESENTATION

Adults:

1. Concussion: headache, dizziness, nausea/vomiting, photophobia/phonophobia, difficulty concentrating, amnesia.

2. Moderate–severe TBI: persistent vomiting, worsening headache, confusion/agitation, focal deficits, seizure,

decreased GCS.

Children:

1. Irritability, lethargy, vomiting, poor feeding, behavior change; infants may present with bulging fontanelle or scalp hematoma.
2. Consider non-accidental trauma in infants/toddlers with inconsistent history.

RED FLAGS

1. GCS <15 at 2 hours post-injury, deteriorating mental status, repeated vomiting.
2. Signs of skull fracture: open/depressed fracture; basilar signs (Battle sign, raccoon eyes, CSF otorrhea/ rhinorrhea).
3. Focal neurological deficit, seizure, unequal pupils.
4. Severe mechanism (high-speed MVC, ejection, fall >1 m child or >1 stair flight adult, struck by high-impact object).
5. Anticoagulant/antiplatelet use or bleeding disorder; age >65; intoxication; persistent severe headache.
6. In children: palpable skull fracture, nonfrontal scalp hematoma (<2 years), abnormal behavior, apnea, suspected NAT.

DIFFERENTIAL DIAGNOSIS

1. Post-concussive symptoms, intracranial hemorrhage (epidural, subdural, SAH), diffuse axonal injury.

2. Cervical spine injury, seizure disorder, syncope, hypoglycemia, intoxication, meningitis.

3. Psychiatric conditions (panic), migraine.

INVESTIGATIONS

Bedside:

1. ABCs, SpO_2, glucose, temperature; serial GCS/ neurologic checks.

2. Cervical spine immobilization until cleared.

Imaging (summarized from open-access guidelines):

1. Adults: Consider CT head within ~1 hour for GCS <13 at presentation or <15 at 2h, suspected open/ depressed skull fracture, any sign of basilar skull fracture, post-traumatic seizure, focal deficit, >1 vomiting episode, or dangerous mechanism. For anticoagulated patients, have low threshold for CT and observation.

2. Children: Use validated rules (e.g., PECARN) — high-risk features include GCS ≤14, palpable skull fracture, altered mental status; intermediate features include loss of consciousness, severe mechanism, severe headache or vomiting (age-dependent). When in doubt, observe 4–6 hours and reassess.

3. CT C-spine if high-risk mechanism or exam; otherwise clinical clearance per validated rules.

MANAGEMENT IN RURAL ER (WITH DRUG DOSAGES)

Primary goals: prevent secondary brain injury, treat life threats, and plan safe disposition/transfer.

Airway & Breathing:

1. Oxygen to maintain SpO_2 ≥ 94%; avoid hypoventilation and severe hyperventilation.
2. If airway compromise or GCS ≤8: RSI with Ketamine 1–2 mg/kg IV (or Etomidate 0.3 mg/kg IV) + Rocuronium 1.2 mg/kg IV. After intubation, target $EtCO_2$ 35–40 mmHg (brief hyperventilation to $EtCO_2$ ~30–35 only if signs of herniation).

Circulation:

1. Avoid hypotension (target SBP ≥110 mmHg adults; age-appropriate pediatric SBP). NS or LR bolus 500–1000 mL (peds 20 mL/kg) as needed.

ICP/Brain Perfusion Measures (if suspected raised ICP: declining GCS, anisocoria, Cushing triad):

1. Head of bed 30°, neutral neck, loosen collar, avoid hypotension/hypoxemia.
2. Hypertonic saline 3%: Adults 2–3 mL/kg IV bolus (or 150 mL over 10–20 min); Pediatrics 3–5 mL/kg IV bolus. May repeat based on clinical response.
3. Mannitol 0.25–1 g/kg IV over 15–20 min (avoid if hypotensive; ensure euvolemia, Foley for diuresis).

Hemostatic therapy:

1. Tranexamic acid (within 3 hours of injury in moderate/ severe TBI or significant head injury): 1 g IV over 10 min, then 1 g IV over 8 hours.

Seizure control/prophylaxis (early post-traumatic seizures):

1. If active seizure: Lorazepam 0.1 mg/kg IV (max 4 mg), may repeat once; then Levetiracetam 60 mg/kg IV (max 4.5 g) OR Phenytoin/Fosphenytoin 20 mg/kg IV.

2. Prophylaxis (severe TBI or cortical contusion/SDH/ EDH): Levetiracetam 20–40 mg/kg IV load (adults commonly 1–1.5 g), then 1 g IV/PO q12h for 7 days (per local protocol).

Symptom control:

1. Analgesia: Acetaminophen 650–1000 mg PO/IV q6h (max 4 g/day). Avoid NSAIDs initially in suspected ICH.

2. Antiemetic: Ondansetron 4–8 mg IV/PO (peds 0.15 mg/kg up to 8 mg).

Concussion-specific care:

1. Cognitive/physical rest 24–48 h, then graded return to school/work and sport per open-access protocols; no same-day return to play.

WHEN TO CALL A SPECIALIST / TRANSFER

1. Any abnormal CT head (ICH, contusion, depressed skull fracture) or deteriorating exam.

2. Persistent GCS <15, focal deficits, seizures, or need for airway/ventilation/ICP therapy.

3. Anticoagulated patients with head injury.

4. Pediatric head injuries with red flags, infants <2 years, suspected NAT.

5. Early contact with neurosurgery/stroke/trauma center; arrange critical care transport if needed.

DISPOSITION

1. Discharge (concussion/mild head injury): normal neuro exam, reliable caregiver, no red flags, improving symptoms, and clear return precautions; provide written concussion advice and gradual return plan.

2. Observe locally: if imaging deferred but risks not zero — observe 4–6 hours with serial exams; admit if symptoms persist/worsen.

3. Transfer: any concern for moderate–severe TBI, need for neurosurgical care, or inability to safely observe.

ADMISSION ORDERS (RURAL HOSPITAL)

1. Monitored bed, neuro checks q1–2h; strict NPO until swallow screen.

2. Head of bed 30°, maintain SBP goals; IV fluids to euvolemia.

3. Hyperosmolar therapy per above if signs of raised ICP; Foley catheter.

4. Seizure prophylaxis if indicated; analgesia/

antiemetic as above.

5. Avoid hypotonic fluids; avoid excessive sedation that impairs neuro exam.

6. Early transfer arrangements if any deterioration or resource limitations.

REFERENCES

1. NICE Guideline NG232 — Head injury: assessment and early management (open): https://www.nice.org.uk/guidance/ng232

2. Emergency Care BC — Minor Head Injury (Canadian CT Head Rule) & Head Injury resources: https://emergencycarebc.ca/clinical_resource

3. Royal Children's Hospital (Melbourne) Clinical Practice Guideline — Head injury (open): https://www.rch.org.au/clinicalguide/guideline_index/Head_injury/

4. Canadian Paediatric Society — Sport-related concussion (open): https://cps.ca/en/documents/position/sport-related-concussion-and-bodychecking

5. CDC HEADS UP — Return to sports/school after concussion (open): https://www.cdc.gov/heads-up/

6. Brain Trauma Foundation — Guidelines for Severe TBI (open): https://braintrauma.org/coma/guidelines/category/Current

7. CRASH-3 Trial (open access summary) — TXA in TBI: https://www.thelancet.com/journals/lancet/article/PIIS0140-6736(19)32233-0/fulltext

DIZZINESS & VERTIGO (CENTRAL VS PERIPHERAL RED FLAGS) — RURAL ER APPROACH

OVERVIEW

Acute dizziness and vertigo are common in rural ERs. Most cases are benign (BPPV, vestibular neuritis), but posterior circulation stroke is a critical 'can't miss'. The goal is to identify central red flags, start symptom control for clearly peripheral conditions, and transfer when stroke is suspected.

CLINICAL PRESENTATION

Patterns help narrow causes:
1. Benign Paroxysmal Positional Vertigo (BPPV): brief (seconds) vertigo triggered by head movement; symptom-free between attacks.
2. Vestibular Neuritis/Labyrinthitis: continuous vertigo for hours–days with nausea/vomiting and spontaneous horizontal nystagmus; hearing loss suggests

labyrinthitis.

3. Vestibular Migraine: episodic vertigo minutes–hours, photophobia/phonophobia, migraine history.

4. Central (e.g., stroke): acute vestibular syndrome with severe imbalance (can't walk unaided), direction-changing or vertical nystagmus, new focal neurologic deficits, severe occipital headache or neck pain.

RED FLAGS (CENTRAL FEATURES)

1. New focal neurological signs: dysarthria, limb ataxia, diplopia, dysphagia, hemiparesis/hemisensory loss.

2. Inability to sit or stand/walk without support (severe truncal ataxia).

3. HINTS exam 'dangerous' findings in continuous vertigo with spontaneous nystagmus: normal head-impulse, direction-changing gaze-evoked nystagmus, or skew deviation.

4. Vertical nystagmus, severe headache/neck pain (consider dissection), new unilateral hearing loss with vertigo (AICA stroke risk), anticoagulation/AFib.

5. Age >60 with vascular risk factors (DM, HTN, prior TIA/stroke).

DIFFERENTIAL DIAGNOSIS

1. Peripheral: BPPV, vestibular neuritis/labyrinthitis, Ménière disease, otitis media.

2. Central: ischemic/hemorrhagic stroke, cerebellitis, MS

relapse, tumor, vertebral/carotid dissection.

3. Other: orthostatic hypotension, anemia, dehydration, medication effects (sedatives, anticonvulsants), hypoglycemia, anxiety/panic.

INVESTIGATIONS

Bedside:

1. ABCs, vitals, glucose, orthostatic BP if presyncope suspected.
2. Full neuro exam; otologic exam for nystagmus and hearing.

Positional testing:

1. Dix–Hallpike for posterior canal BPPV (classic torsional up-beating nystagmus).
2. Supine roll test for horizontal canal BPPV.
3. HINTS (only for continuous vertigo with spontaneous nystagmus and no obvious focal deficits; requires training): head-impulse, nystagmus, test of skew. Any 'central' sign → manage as stroke.

Imaging:

1. If central signs or high suspicion: urgent neuroimaging/ transfer. Non-contrast CT can exclude hemorrhage; MRI with diffusion is most sensitive for posterior stroke (often not available rurally). Consider CTA head/neck if dissection suspected.

MANAGEMENT IN RURAL ER (WITH DRUG DOSAGES)

For clear peripheral causes:

1. BPPV: perform canalith repositioning (Epley) — avoid vestibular suppressants after first 24–48 h; provide home Epley handout.

2. Vestibular neuritis/labyrinthitis: short course vestibular suppressants/antiemetics for severe symptoms (limit to 48–72 h to promote compensation):

   ⇒ - Dimenhydrinate 50 mg PO/IV/IM q6h PRN (peds 1–2 mg/kg/dose q6h, max 50 mg).

   ⇒ - Meclizine 25–50 mg PO q6–8h PRN (adults).

   ⇒ - Diazepam 2–5 mg PO/IV q6–8h PRN or Lorazepam 0.5–1 mg PO/IV q6h PRN (use sparingly; fall risk).

   ⇒ - Ondansetron 4–8 mg IV/PO q6–8h PRN (peds 0.15 mg/kg up to 8 mg).

   ⇒ - Metoclopramide 10 mg IV/PO q6–8h PRN (peds 0.1–0.15 mg/kg; max 10 mg), +/- Diphenhydramine 25–50 mg IV to reduce akathisia.

3. Consider corticosteroids for vestibular neuritis within 72 h (evidence mixed): Prednisone 60 mg PO daily ×5 days, then taper by 10 mg/day over 5 days.

4. Hydration: IV crystalloids for persistent emesis.

If central features or stroke suspected:

1. Treat per stroke pathway (see Stroke chapter): maintain SpO_2 ≥94%, permissive hypertension unless tPA candidates, check glucose, avoid excessive sedation, urgent transfer for imaging/thrombolysis/thrombectomy.
2. If vertebral/carotid dissection suspected with neuro deficits: prioritize CTA and stroke-center transfer.

Vestibular migraine (if typical phenotype and no central signs):

1. Acute therapy as per migraine protocols: Metoclopramide 10 mg IV + Diphenhydramine 25 mg IV; Ketorolac 15–30 mg IV if no contraindication; Magnesium sulfate 1–2 g IV over 20–30 min.

WHEN TO CALL A SPECIALIST / TRANSFER

1. Any central red flag or abnormal HINTS, new focal neuro deficits, severe gait/truncal ataxia, new unilateral hearing loss, sudden severe headache/neck pain (dissection), anticoagulation/AFib with acute vestibular syndrome.
2. Persistent vomiting/dehydration or inability to ambulate safely despite therapy.
3. Children with atypical or severe presentations.
4. Early neurology/otolaryngology consultation and transfer to stroke-capable center if concern for posterior stroke.

DISPOSITION

1. Discharge: classic BPPV improved after Epley;
    vestibular neuritis with improving symptoms, tolerating
    PO, safe ambulation, reliable follow-up; provide return
    precautions and self-Epley instructions.
2. Observe locally: diagnostic uncertainty, need for
    repeated antiemetics/IV fluids.
3. Transfer: any central features, need for MRI/CTA
    not available, or worsening symptoms.

ADMISSION ORDERS (RURAL HOSPITAL)

1. Monitored bed if high fall risk; neuro checks.
2. IV fluids if dehydrated; antiemetics/suppressants short
    term as above.
3. Early mobilization and vestibular rehab exercises
    once stable.
4. If stroke suspected: follow stroke orders (tele-
    stroke consult, imaging, permissive BP, NPO until
    swallow screen).

REFERENCES

1. Emergency Care BC — Vertigo/Acute Vestibular
    Syndrome & HINTS resources: https://
    emergencycarebc.ca/clinical_resource
2. AAFP — Dizziness: Approach to Evaluation and
    Management (open): https://www.aafp.org
3. Canadian Stroke Best Practices — Posterior
    circulation stroke recognition: https://www.

strokebestpractices.ca

4. NICE CKS — Vertigo; Labyrinthitis/Vestibular
    neuritis (open): https://cks.nice.org.uk

5. CoreEM — HINTS Exam, Acute Vestibular
    Syndrome (open): https://coreem.net

6. CDC Stroke — general stroke recognition: https://
    www.cdc.gov/stroke

SECTION V –
ABDOMINAL &
GASTROINTESTINAL
EMERGENCIES

ACUTE ABDOMINAL PAIN (RED FLAGS IN RURAL ER) — RURAL ER APPROACH

OVERVIEW

Acute abdominal pain is a common rural ER presentation with causes ranging from benign to immediately life-threatening. Resource limitations require early identification of red flags, stabilization, and timely transfer when necessary. Initial priorities are rapid assessment, pain control, ruling out surgical emergencies, and arranging appropriate imaging or transfer.

CLINICAL PRESENTATION

1. Pain characteristics: onset, location, radiation, severity, progression.
2. Associated symptoms: nausea, vomiting, diarrhea, constipation, fever, urinary or gynecological symptoms.
3. In children: irritability, poor feeding, inconsolable crying, lethargy.
4. Elderly: may have vague or minimal symptoms despite severe disease.

RED FLAGS

1. Hemodynamic instability: hypotension, tachycardia, shock.

2. Severe sudden onset pain ('pain out of proportion' → mesenteric ischemia).

3. Peritonitis: rebound tenderness, guarding, rigidity.

4. GI bleeding: hematemesis, melena, hematochezia.

5. Abdominal aortic aneurysm (AAA) suspicion: pulsatile mass, hypotension, back/flank pain, elderly male.

6. Bowel obstruction: bilious vomiting, abdominal distension, absent bowel movements.

7. Pregnant patient: ectopic pregnancy, abruption, ruptured uterus.

8. Pediatric red flags: bilious vomiting, currant jelly stool (intussusception), abdominal mass, lethargy.

DIFFERENTIAL DIAGNOSIS

1. Surgical: appendicitis, cholecystitis, perforated viscus, bowel obstruction, AAA, mesenteric ischemia.

2. Medical: gastroenteritis, pancreatitis, hepatitis, renal colic, pyelonephritis, DKA.

3. Gynecologic/obstetric: ectopic pregnancy, ovarian torsion, PID, abruption.

4. Pediatric: intussusception, malrotation/volvulus, incarcerated hernia.

INVESTIGATIONS

1. Bedside: vitals, SpO_2, urine dip (infection, hematuria, pregnancy test in all females of childbearing age).

2. Labs: CBC, electrolytes, creatinine, LFTs, lipase, lactate, troponin if chest pain overlap, beta-hCG in women.

3. Imaging: bedside ultrasound (FAST, AAA, gallbladder, hydronephrosis, free fluid); X-ray for obstruction or perforation (free air); CT abdomen/pelvis if available and stable.

MANAGEMENT IN RURAL ER (WITH DRUG DOSAGES)

Stabilization:

1. IV access ×2 large bore.

2. Oxygen if SpO_2 < 94%.

3. IV fluids: NS or LR bolus 500–1000 mL (peds 20 mL/kg) for shock/dehydration.

Analgesia:

1. Morphine 0.05–0.1 mg/kg IV q2–4h PRN (adults typical 2–5 mg IV).

2. Fentanyl 0.5–1 mcg/kg IV q30–60min PRN (adults typical 25–50 mcg).

3. Acetaminophen 650–1000 mg PO/IV q6h (peds 15 mg/kg q6h).

Antiemetics:

1. Ondansetron 4–8 mg IV/PO q6–8h (peds 0.15 mg/kg up to 8 mg).
2. Metoclopramide 10 mg IV/PO q6–8h (peds 0.1–0.15 mg/kg).

Antibiotics (for suspected intra-abdominal infection/ peritonitis):

1. Ceftriaxone 2 g IV daily + Metronidazole 500 mg IV q8h.
2. Pediatric: Ceftriaxone 50 mg/kg IV daily (max 2 g) + Metronidazole 10 mg/kg IV q8h.

Special cases:

1. Suspected AAA rupture: permissive hypotension (SBP 80–100) until surgical control.
2. Suspected ectopic pregnancy: IV fluids, O-negative blood if unstable; urgent transfer.
3. Pediatric intussusception: IV fluids, NG decompression, urgent transfer for reduction.

WHEN TO CALL A SPECIALIST / TRANSFER

1. All unstable patients.
2. Suspected AAA, mesenteric ischemia, bowel perforation, or peritonitis.
3. Pediatric surgical emergencies (intussusception, malrotation, appendicitis with sepsis).
4. Pregnant patients with abdominal pain and red flags.
5. If imaging unavailable and diagnosis uncertain but

concern for surgical pathology.

DISPOSITION

1. Discharge: only if benign exam, no red flags, tolerating PO, reliable follow-up.
2. Admit locally: mild/moderate illness with available diagnostics and monitoring.
3. Transfer: most surgical emergencies, unstable patients, pediatric or pregnant patients with concerning features.

ADMISSION ORDERS (RURAL HOSPITAL)

1. Admit to monitored bed if unstable.
2. IV fluids as needed, strict I&O.
3. Analgesia and antiemetics as above.
4. NPO, NG tube if obstruction suspected.
5. IV antibiotics if infection suspected.
6. Serial abdominal exams.
7. Prepare for transfer if deterioration.

REFERENCES

1. Emergency Care BC — Abdominal Pain & Surgical Emergencies: https://emergencycarebc.ca/clinical_resource
2. NICE CKS — Abdominal Pain (open): https://cks.nice.org.uk
3. Canadian Paediatric Society — Acute Abdominal Pain in Children: https://cps.ca

4. CDC Abdominal Aortic Aneurysm Resources: https://www.cdc.gov
5. WHO Emergency & Surgical Care Guidance: https://www.who.int

GASTROINTESTINAL BLEEDING (UPPER VS LOWER) — RURAL ER APPROACH

OVERVIEW

Gastrointestinal (GI) bleeding is a potentially life-threatening emergency. It may present as hematemesis, melena, or hematochezia. In rural ERs, priorities include rapid resuscitation, localization (upper vs lower), early pharmacologic therapy, and stabilization for transfer to endoscopy-capable centers.

CLINICAL PRESENTATION

1. Upper GI bleed: hematemesis (bright red or coffee ground), melena, epigastric pain.
2. Lower GI bleed: hematochezia, maroon stools, abdominal cramps.
3. Massive UGIB may also cause hematochezia if rapid transit.
4. Associated features: hypotension, tachycardia, syncope, pallor, shock.
5. Pediatric: swallowed maternal blood (newborn),

Meckel's diverticulum, intussusception.

RED FLAGS

1. Hemodynamic instability: hypotension, tachycardia, shock.
2. Hematemesis or large-volume hematochezia.
3. Syncope, altered LOC.
4. Known varices, cirrhosis, anticoagulant use.
5. Age >60, comorbidities (cardiac disease, renal failure).

DIFFERENTIAL DIAGNOSIS

1. Upper GI causes: peptic ulcer disease, gastritis, esophageal varices, Mallory–Weiss tear.
2. Lower GI causes: diverticulosis, angiodysplasia, colorectal cancer, IBD, hemorrhoids, anal fissure.
3. Other: swallowed blood (epistaxis), small bowel bleeding.

INVESTIGATIONS

Bedside:

1. Vitals, SpO_2, orthostatic BP.
2. NG/OG tube aspiration if uncertain source (blood suggests UGIB).

Labs:

1. CBC, type & crossmatch, INR/PTT, electrolytes, creatinine, liver function tests.

2. Consider troponin if chest pain or shock.

Imaging:

1. CXR if concern for aspiration or perforation.
2. CT angiography if massive LGIB and available.

MANAGEMENT IN RURAL ER (WITH DRUG DOSAGES)

Stabilization:

1. 2 large-bore IVs, oxygen to keep $SpO_2 \geq 94\%$.
2. IV fluids: NS or LR bolus 500–1000 mL (peds 20 mL/kg). Avoid over-resuscitation in variceal bleed.
3. Blood transfusion if Hb <70 g/L (restrictive) or <90 g/L in ongoing bleeding/cardiac disease.
4. Massive transfusion protocol if unstable.

Pharmacologic therapy:

1. Proton Pump Inhibitor (PPI): Pantoprazole 80 mg IV bolus, then 8 mg/hr infusion; Pediatrics: 1 mg/kg IV bolus then 0.1 mg/kg/hr infusion.
2. Variceal bleed: Octreotide 50 mcg IV bolus, then 50 mcg/hr infusion.
3. Antibiotics (cirrhotics/variceal bleed): Ceftriaxone 1 g IV daily; Pediatrics: 50 mg/kg IV daily (max 2 g).
4. Correct coagulopathy: Vitamin K 10 mg IV; consider PCC 25–50 units/kg IV if on warfarin with active bleed.

Adjuncts:

1. NG/OG suction if hematemesis.
2. Avoid NSAIDs/anticoagulants where possible.
3. Consider tranexamic acid (TXA) 1 g IV over 10 min then 1 g IV over 8 h (evidence mixed).

WHEN TO CALL A SPECIALIST / TRANSFER

1. All cases with hemodynamic instability or ongoing bleeding.
2. Variceal bleed (needs endoscopy, possible TIPS).
3. Pediatric GI bleeds (require pediatric gastroenterology).
4. Transfer if endoscopy unavailable locally or if massive bleed.

DISPOSITION

1. Discharge: only if minor bleed, stable, benign source (e.g., hemorrhoid, anal fissure) with follow-up.
2. Admit locally: moderate bleed, stable, responding to therapy.
3. Transfer: unstable, variceal bleed, massive ongoing hemorrhage, pediatric unstable cases.

ADMISSION ORDERS (RURAL HOSPITAL)

1. Admit to monitored bed.
2. Serial Hb q6–8h, type & screen.
3. Pantoprazole infusion; Octreotide if variceal.
4. NPO; IV fluids/blood products as required.

5. Monitor vitals q15–30min initially.

6. Prepare for transfer if unstable or worsening.

REFERENCES

1. Emergency Care BC — Upper GI Bleed & Lower GI Bleed resources: https://emergencycarebc.ca/clinical_resource

2. NICE CKS — GI bleeding (upper & lower): https://cks.nice.org.uk

3. CDC — Gastrointestinal Bleeding (public health/epidemiology): https://www.cdc.gov

4. WHO Emergency & Surgical Care Guidance: https://www.who.int

BOWEL OBSTRUCTION & PERFORATION SUSPICION — RURAL ER APPROACH

OVERVIEW

Bowel obstruction and perforated viscus are surgical emergencies with high morbidity and mortality. In rural ERs, priorities are rapid recognition, resuscitation, early antibiotics, NG decompression, and transfer for definitive surgical management if resources are limited.

CLINICAL PRESENTATION

Bowel Obstruction:
1. Colicky abdominal pain, vomiting (bilious/feculent), abdominal distension, constipation/obstipation.
2. High-pitched or absent bowel sounds.

Perforation:
1. Sudden severe abdominal pain, peritonitis (rigidity, rebound tenderness, guarding).
2. Fever, tachycardia, hypotension, septic shock.
3. History of peptic ulcer disease, diverticulitis,

trauma, recent surgery.

RED FLAGS

1. Hemodynamic instability.
2. Signs of peritonitis (rigidity, rebound, severe tenderness).
3. Persistent vomiting with electrolyte abnormalities.
4. Absent bowel sounds with sepsis/shock.
5. Free air on imaging (suggests perforation).

DIFFERENTIAL DIAGNOSIS

1. Bowel obstruction: adhesions, hernia, malignancy, volvulus, Crohn's strictures.
2. Perforation: peptic ulcer, diverticulitis, ischemic bowel, trauma, malignancy.
3. Other mimics: gastroenteritis, severe pancreatitis, mesenteric ischemia.

INVESTIGATIONS

Bedside:

1. Vitals, SpO_2, urine output, bedside glucose.

Labs:

1. CBC, electrolytes, creatinine, LFTs, lipase, lactate (ischemia), coagulation profile, type & crossmatch.

Imaging:

1. Upright CXR/AXR: free air under diaphragm

(perforation), dilated loops, air-fluid levels (obstruction).

2. POCUS: free fluid, peristalsis, dilated loops.
3. CT abdomen/pelvis with contrast (if available) for confirmation and surgical planning.

MANAGEMENT IN RURAL ER (WITH DRUG DOSAGES)

Stabilization:

1. ABCs, 2 large-bore IVs.
2. Oxygen to maintain $SpO_2 \geq 94\%$.
3. IV fluids: NS/LR bolus 500–1000 mL (peds 20 mL/kg), then reassess.
4. Insert NG tube for decompression (suction).
5. Foley catheter for urine output.

Analgesia:

1. Morphine 0.05–0.1 mg/kg IV q2–4h PRN (adults 2–5 mg typical).
2. Fentanyl 0.5–1 mcg/kg IV q30–60min PRN (adults 25–50 mcg typical).
3. Acetaminophen 650–1000 mg PO/IV q6h (peds 15 mg/kg q6h).

Antibiotics (for suspected perforation/peritonitis or strangulated obstruction):

1. Ceftriaxone 2 g IV daily + Metronidazole 500 mg IV q8h.

2. Pediatrics: Ceftriaxone 50 mg/kg IV daily (max 2 g) + Metronidazole 10 mg/kg IV q8h.

Adjuncts:

1. Correct electrolytes (esp. K+, Mg2+).
2. Broad-spectrum antibiotics before transfer if perforation suspected.
3. Vasopressors if persistent hypotension despite fluids (Norepinephrine 2–20 mcg/min IV).

WHEN TO CALL A SPECIALIST / TRANSFER

1. All suspected perforations.
2. Complete obstruction, strangulation, ischemia.
3. Hemodynamic instability or sepsis.
4. Pediatric obstruction (intussusception, malrotation).
5. Pregnant patient with obstruction/peritonitis.

DISPOSITION

1. Discharge: NOT appropriate if obstruction or perforation suspected.
2. Admit locally: only partial obstruction, stable, if surgical support available.
3. Transfer: most cases with complete obstruction, suspected perforation, ischemia, or no local surgical capacity.

ADMISSION ORDERS (RURAL HOSPITAL)

1. NPO, NG decompression, IV fluids, Foley catheter.
2. IV antibiotics if infection suspected.
3. Analgesia and antiemetics.
4. Serial abdominal exams, monitor vitals and urine output.
5. Prepare for urgent transfer if worsening.

REFERENCES

1. Emergency Care BC — Bowel Obstruction, Perforation: https://emergencycarebc.ca/clinical_resource
2. NICE CKS — Abdominal Pain/Perforation/Obstruction: https://cks.nice.org.uk
3. Canadian Association of General Surgeons (open resources): https://cags-accg.ca
4. CDC — Abdominal Emergencies/Public Health: https://www.cdc.gov
5. WHO Emergency & Surgical Care Guidance: https://www.who.int

PEDIATRIC ABDOMINAL EMERGENCIES (APPENDICITIS, INTUSSUSCEPTION) — RURAL ER APPROACH

OVERVIEW

Pediatric abdominal pain is a frequent challenge in rural ERs. Appendicitis is the most common surgical emergency, while intussusception is the leading cause of bowel obstruction in infants and toddlers. Prompt recognition, supportive care, and early transfer when surgery or advanced imaging is needed are critical.

CLINICAL PRESENTATION

Appendicitis:
1. Periumbilical pain migrating to right lower quadrant.
2. Anorexia, nausea/vomiting, low-grade fever.
3. RLQ tenderness, rebound, guarding.
4. In infants/young children: irritability, poor feeding, lethargy.

Intussusception:

1. Intermittent colicky abdominal pain with episodes of crying/drawing knees up.
2. Vomiting (may be bilious), lethargy between episodes.
3. 'Currant jelly' stool (blood + mucus).
4. Sausage-shaped abdominal mass, distension.
5. May progress to shock/perforation if delayed.

RED FLAGS

1. Hemodynamic instability or shock.
2. Signs of peritonitis (rigidity, rebound tenderness).
3. Bilious vomiting in infants/children.
4. Currant jelly stool (suggests intussusception).
5. Persistent lethargy, altered LOC.
6. Palpable mass or abdominal distension with pain.

DIFFERENTIAL DIAGNOSIS

1. Gastroenteritis.
2. Mesenteric adenitis.
3. UTI/pyelonephritis.
4. Constipation.
5. Malrotation with volvulus.
6. In females: ovarian torsion, PID, ectopic pregnancy (adolescents).

INVESTIGATIONS

1. Bedside: vitals, urine dip, pregnancy test in adolescent

females.

2. Labs: CBC, electrolytes, CRP, type & screen if surgery anticipated.

3. Imaging: ultrasound is preferred (appendix visualization, 'target sign' for intussusception).

4. AXR: may show obstruction, perforation, or mass in intussusception.

5. CT abdomen/pelvis only if diagnosis uncertain and available (avoid routine in children).

MANAGEMENT IN RURAL ER (WITH DRUG DOSAGES)

Stabilization:

1. IV access, fluids: NS/LR bolus 20 mL/kg for dehydration/shock.

2. Oxygen if hypoxemic.

3. NPO, NG decompression if persistent vomiting/ obstruction suspected.

Analgesia:

1. Morphine 0.05–0.1 mg/kg IV q2–4h PRN.

2. Acetaminophen 15 mg/kg PO/IV q6h (max 75 mg/kg/ day).

3. Ibuprofen 10 mg/kg PO q6–8h (if >6 months old).

Antibiotics (if perforation or peritonitis suspected):

1. Ceftriaxone 50 mg/kg IV daily (max 2 g) + Metronidazole 10 mg/kg IV q8h.

2. Alternative: Ampicillin 50 mg/kg IV q6h + Gentamicin 5 mg/kg IV daily + Metronidazole 10 mg/kg IV q8h.

Intussusception-specific:

1. IV fluids and stabilization first.
2. Do NOT delay transfer for enema reduction if unstable or peritonitis present.
3. If stable and resources available: air/contrast enema may be diagnostic and therapeutic (performed in pediatric centers).

WHEN TO CALL A SPECIALIST / TRANSFER

1. All suspected appendicitis or intussusception.
2. Shock, peritonitis, or perforation — urgent surgical transfer.
3. If enema reduction not available locally.
4. Infants <1 year with bilious vomiting or abdominal distension (possible malrotation/volvulus).

DISPOSITION

1. Discharge: NOT appropriate if appendicitis or intussusception suspected.
2. Admit locally: only if diagnosis confirmed and surgical backup available.
3. Transfer: most suspected cases requiring surgery or advanced pediatric intervention.

ADMISSION ORDERS (RURAL HOSPITAL)

1. NPO, IV fluids, NG decompression if needed.
2. IV antibiotics if infection suspected.
3. Analgesia and antipyretics as above.
4. Serial abdominal exams.
5. Prepare for urgent transfer if diagnosis confirmed/ suspected.

REFERENCES

1. Canadian Paediatric Society — Acute Abdominal Pain & Intussusception: https://cps.ca
2. Emergency Care BC — Pediatric Appendicitis/ Intussusception: https://emergencycarebc.ca/clinical_ resource
3. NICE CKS — Abdominal Pain in Children, Appendicitis: https://cks.nice.org.uk
4. CDC — Pediatric Abdominal Pain/Emergencies (public health resources): https://www.cdc.gov
5. WHO Emergency & Surgical Care Guidance: https://www.who.int

SECTION VI – RENAL & UROLOGIC EMERGENCIES

RENAL COLIC & KIDNEY STONES — RURAL ER APPROACH

OVERVIEW

Renal colic, most often due to kidney stones, is a common and extremely painful presentation in rural ERs. Most stones pass spontaneously, but the key priorities are ruling out obstructive uropathy, infection (obstructed infected kidney = urologic emergency), and providing effective analgesia and hydration. Definitive stone management (lithotripsy, surgery) is usually unavailable in rural settings, making stabilization and transfer decisions essential.

CLINICAL PRESENTATION

1. Sudden, severe flank pain radiating to groin/testicle/labia.
2. Restlessness, constant movement (unable to find position of comfort).
3. Nausea, vomiting.
4. Hematuria (gross or microscopic).
5. +/- fever (red flag for infected obstruction).

6. Pediatric: may present with irritability, abdominal pain, vomiting.

RED FLAGS

1. Fever with flank pain (obstructed infected kidney/ pyonephrosis → emergency).
2. Solitary kidney or known chronic kidney disease.
3. Intractable vomiting or uncontrolled pain.
4. Anuria or bilateral obstruction.
5. Signs of sepsis (tachycardia, hypotension, altered LOC).

DIFFERENTIAL DIAGNOSIS

1. Pyelonephritis.
2. Abdominal aortic aneurysm (elderly with atypical presentation).
3. Biliary colic, appendicitis, diverticulitis.
4. Ovarian torsion, ectopic pregnancy (women of childbearing age).

INVESTIGATIONS

1. Bedside: vitals, urine dip (hematuria, infection, nitrites/ leukocytes), pregnancy test in women.
2. Labs: CBC, electrolytes, creatinine, urinalysis & culture.
3. Imaging: POCUS (hydronephrosis, stone if visible); non-contrast CT KUB is gold standard if available; KUB X-ray may detect radiopaque stones;

Ultrasound preferred in pregnancy/pediatrics.

MANAGEMENT IN RURAL ER (WITH DRUG DOSAGES)

Analgesia (first-line):

1. NSAIDs: Ketorolac 30 mg IV/IM q6h PRN (max 120 mg/day); Pediatrics: 0.5 mg/kg IV/IM q6h (max 30 mg/ dose).
2. If NSAID contraindicated: Morphine 0.05–0.1 mg/kg IV q2–4h PRN (adults 2–5 mg typical).
3. Fentanyl 25–50 mcg IV q30–60min PRN.
4. Acetaminophen 650–1000 mg PO/IV q6h (peds 15 mg/kg q6h).

Adjuncts:

1. IV fluids: NS 500–1000 mL bolus, then maintenance (not for stone passage but for hydration).
2. Antiemetics: Ondansetron 4–8 mg IV/PO q6–8h (peds 0.15 mg/kg up to 8 mg).
3. Tamsulosin 0.4 mg PO daily may help stone passage (>5 mm, distal ureter).

If infection suspected (obstructed infected stone = emergency):

1. IV antibiotics: Ceftriaxone 2 g IV daily; Pediatrics: 50 mg/kg IV daily (max 2 g).
2. Early urology consultation/transfer for decompression (stent/nephrostomy).

If impending sepsis/shock:

1. Broad-spectrum antibiotics (Ceftriaxone + Gentamicin or Piperacillin–Tazobactam if available).
2. Vasopressors if hypotension persists (Norepinephrine 2–20 mcg/min IV).

WHEN TO CALL A SPECIALIST / TRANSFER

1. Obstructed infected kidney (fever, sepsis, obstruction).
2. Solitary kidney, rising creatinine, anuria.
3. Large stone unlikely to pass (>10 mm) or persistent obstruction.
4. Uncontrolled pain or vomiting despite therapy.
5. Pediatric or pregnant patient with obstruction.

DISPOSITION

1. Discharge: if pain controlled, tolerating PO, normal renal function, no infection, and reliable follow-up.
2. Admit locally: if moderate pain, unable to discharge safely, or awaiting transfer.
3. Transfer: all cases with infection, obstruction, solitary kidney, or uncontrolled symptoms.

ADMISSION ORDERS (RURAL HOSPITAL)

1. Admit to monitored bed if unstable.
2. IV fluids and urine output monitoring.
3. Analgesia and antiemetics as above.
4. NPO if surgical intervention likely.

5. IV antibiotics if infection suspected.

6. Prepare for transfer if criteria met.

REFERENCES

1. Emergency Care BC — Renal Colic & Kidney Stones: https://emergencycarebc.ca/clinical_resource

2. NICE CKS — Renal Colic: https://cks.nice.org.uk

3. Canadian Urological Association (CUA) Guidelines — Kidney Stones (open summaries): https://www.cua.org

4. CDC Kidney Disease Resources: https://www.cdc.gov

5. WHO Emergency & Surgical Care Guidance: https://www.who.int

HYPERKALEMIA & HYPOKALEMIA (RURAL ER APPROACH)

OVERVIEW

Electrolyte disturbances, especially potassium abnormalities, are life-threatening if unrecognized. Hyperkalemia can cause lethal arrhythmias, while hypokalemia predisposes to arrhythmias and muscle weakness. In rural ERs, prompt recognition, ECG monitoring, temporizing therapy, and safe transfer are critical.

CLINICAL PRESENTATION

Hyperkalemia:
1. Weakness, fatigue, paresthesias.
2. ECG: peaked T waves, widened QRS, sine wave, ventricular arrhythmias, asystole.

Hypokalemia:
1. Weakness, cramps, ileus, constipation.
2. ECG: flattened T waves, U waves, ST depression, arrhythmias (VT, VF).

RED FLAGS

1. K+ ≥6.5 mmol/L (or rapidly rising).
2. ECG changes (any level).
3. Hemodynamic instability.
4. Severe hypokalemia (K+ <2.5 mmol/L).
5. Arrhythmias or neuromuscular weakness (respiratory failure risk).

DIFFERENTIAL DIAGNOSIS

1. Hyperkalemia: renal failure, rhabdomyolysis, hemolysis, tumor lysis, ACE inhibitors, potassium-sparing diuretics.
2. Hypokalemia: diuretics, vomiting, diarrhea, hyperaldosteronism, insulin therapy, beta-agonists.

INVESTIGATIONS

1. Labs: electrolytes, renal function, CBC.
2. ECG: assess for potassium-related changes.
3. Consider repeat sample (exclude pseudohyperkalemia from hemolyzed sample).

MANAGEMENT IN RURAL ER (WITH DRUG DOSAGES)

Hyperkalemia (K+ ≥6.0 mmol/L or with ECG changes):

1. Cardiac stabilization:
2. Calcium gluconate 10%: 10 mL IV over 2–5 min; may repeat in 5–10 min if no ECG improvement. (Peds: 0.5

mL/kg IV, max 10 mL).

Shift potassium into cells:

1. Insulin + Dextrose: Regular insulin 10 units IV + D50W 25 g IV (50 mL) over 15–30 min; Peds: 0.1 units/kg insulin IV + 0.5 g/kg dextrose IV.

2. Salbutamol: 10–20 mg nebulized over 10 min; Peds: 0.15 mg/kg (max 10 mg).

3. Sodium bicarbonate: 50 mEq IV over 5 min (use in metabolic acidosis).

Remove potassium:

1. Furosemide 20–40 mg IV (if volume replete, normal renal function).

2. Kayexalate (sodium polystyrene sulfonate) 15–30 g PO/PR (rarely used, slow onset).

3. Dialysis: definitive in severe/renal failure (requires transfer).

Hypokalemia:

1. 1. Mild (K+ 3.0–3.5, asymptomatic):

2. Oral potassium chloride 20–40 mEq PO.

Moderate (K+ 2.5–3.0, symptoms or ECG changes):

1. Oral KCl 40–60 mEq PO in divided doses.

2. IV replacement if unable PO: 10–20 mEq KCl in 100 mL NS over 1 h (max 40 mEq/4 h).

3. Peds: 0.5–1 mEq/kg per dose IV (max 40 mEq).

Severe (K+ <2.5 or symptomatic):

1. IV KCl via central line if available, 20–40 mEq/h with continuous ECG monitoring.
2. Correct magnesium if low: MgSO4 2 g IV over 1 h (peds: 25–50 mg/kg, max 2 g).

Monitor:
1. ECG monitoring during replacement.
2. Recheck K+ q2–4h in acute cases.

WHEN TO CALL A SPECIALIST / TRANSFER

1. Hyperkalemia with ECG changes or K+ ≥6.5.
2. Hypokalemia <2.5 or with arrhythmias.
3. All patients needing dialysis.
4. Pediatric patients with severe derangements.

DISPOSITION

1. Discharge: mild, corrected in ER, no underlying disease, reliable follow-up.
2. Admit locally: moderate abnormalities requiring monitoring.
3. Transfer: severe or refractory cases, dialysis requirement, unstable patients.

ADMISSION ORDERS (RURAL HOSPITAL)

1. Admit to monitored bed with ECG.
2. Serial potassium monitoring.
3. Replace K+ orally/IV as indicated.
4. Treat underlying cause.

5. Prepare for transfer if unstable or refractory.

REFERENCES

1. Emergency Care BC — Hyperkalemia & Hypokalemia: https://emergencycarebc.ca/clinical_resource

2. NICE CKS — Electrolyte Disturbances: https://cks. nice.org.uk

3. Canadian Society of Nephrology (open guidance): https://www.csnscn.ca

4. CDC Potassium & Renal Health Resources: https://www.cdc.gov

5. WHO Emergency & Critical Care Guidance: https://www.who.int

ELECTROLYTE DISTURBANCES — HYPERCALCEMIA & HYPOCALCEMIA (RURAL ER APPROACH)

OVERVIEW

Calcium abnormalities can present with life-threatening complications. Hypercalcemia is often due to malignancy or hyperparathyroidism, while hypocalcemia may follow thyroid/parathyroid surgery, sepsis, or renal failure. Both conditions may cause arrhythmias and seizures, requiring urgent stabilization in the rural ER.

CLINICAL PRESENTATION

Hypercalcemia:
1. Polyuria, polydipsia, dehydration.
2. Nausea, vomiting, constipation, abdominal pain.
3. Weakness, confusion, altered LOC.
4. Severe: arrhythmias, coma.

Hypocalcemia:

1. Paresthesias, muscle cramps, carpopedal spasm, tetany.
2. Chvostek and Trousseau signs.
3. Seizures, laryngospasm.
4. ECG: prolonged QT interval.

RED FLAGS

1. Hypercalcemia >3.5 mmol/L (14 mg/dL).
2. Hypocalcemia <1.8 mmol/L (7 mg/dL).
3. Arrhythmias or seizures.
4. Severe dehydration or shock.
5. Altered mental status or coma.

DIFFERENTIAL DIAGNOSIS

Hypercalcemia: primary hyperparathyroidism, malignancy (PTHrP, bone mets), thiazides, vitamin D toxicity, sarcoidosis.

Hypocalcemia: post-thyroid/parathyroid surgery, CKD, hypomagnesemia, sepsis, pancreatitis, tumor lysis, medications (bisphosphonates, cisplatin).

INVESTIGATIONS

1. Serum calcium (corrected for albumin), ionized calcium.
2. Magnesium, phosphate, renal function.
3. PTH, vitamin D levels if available.
4. ECG: shortened QT (hypercalcemia), prolonged

QT (hypocalcemia).

MANAGEMENT IN RURAL ER (WITH DRUG DOSAGES)

Hypercalcemia:

1. IV fluids: NS 1–2 L bolus then 150–200 mL/hr (peds 20 mL/kg bolus, then maintenance).
2. Loop diuretic (after fluids, only if volume overload): Furosemide 20–40 mg IV (peds 1 mg/kg, max 20 mg).
3. Calcitonin 4 IU/kg IM/SC q12h (short-term bridge).
4. Bisphosphonates (if available, for malignancy-associated): Zoledronic acid 4 mg IV over 15 min or Pamidronate 60–90 mg IV over 2–4 h.
5. Dialysis if refractory or severe renal failure.

Hypocalcemia:

1. IV calcium gluconate 10%: 10–20 mL (1–2 g) in 50–100 mL D5W over 10 min; may repeat q10 min if symptomatic.
2. Continuous infusion: 100 mL of 10% calcium gluconate in 1 L D5W or NS, run at 50–100 mL/hr (titrate to ionized calcium).
3. Pediatrics: 0.5 mL/kg of 10% calcium gluconate (max 10 mL) IV over 10 min with cardiac monitoring.
4. Correct magnesium if low: MgSO4 2 g IV over 30 min (peds 25–50 mg/kg, max 2 g).
5. Oral calcium: Calcium carbonate 500–1000 mg PO TID once stable.

6. Vitamin D supplementation if deficiency-related.

WHEN TO CALL A SPECIALIST / TRANSFER

1. Hypercalcemia >3.5 mmol/L or refractory to fluids.
2. Hypocalcemia with seizures, tetany, laryngospasm, or arrhythmias.
3. All pediatric cases with severe derangements.
4. Patients requiring dialysis or bisphosphonate infusion not available locally.

DISPOSITION

1. Discharge: mild cases corrected and stable, underlying cause addressed.
2. Admit locally: moderate cases requiring IV replacement/monitoring.
3. Transfer: severe or refractory cases, unstable patients, need for dialysis or ICU care.

ADMISSION ORDERS (RURAL HOSPITAL)

1. Admit to monitored bed with ECG.
2. Serial calcium and electrolyte checks q4–6h.
3. IV fluids, calcium replacement or lowering therapy as indicated.
4. Seizure precautions for hypocalcemia.
5. Strict I&O, monitor urine output.

REFERENCES

1. Emergency Care BC — Hypercalcemia &

Hypocalcemia: https://emergencycarebc.ca/clinical_ resource

2. NICE CKS — Calcium Disorders: https://cks.nice.org. uk

3. Canadian Society of Nephrology — Calcium Disorders (open summaries): https://www.csnscn.ca

4. CDC Calcium & Bone Health Resources: https:// www.cdc.gov

5. WHO Emergency & Critical Care Guidance: https://www.who.int

ELECTROLYTE DISTURBANCES — HYPONATREMIA & HYPERNATREMIA (RURAL ER APPROACH)

OVERVIEW

Sodium abnormalities are common and can be life-threatening. Hyponatremia can cause seizures and cerebral edema, while hypernatremia can lead to brain shrinkage, hemorrhage, and death. In rural ERs, focus on identifying underlying causes, correcting sodium safely, and arranging transfer if severe.

CLINICAL PRESENTATION

Hyponatremia:
1. Mild: nausea, headache, confusion.
2. Moderate–severe: vomiting, lethargy, seizures, coma.
3. Often associated with diuretics, heart failure, cirrhosis, SIADH, vomiting/diarrhea.

Hypernatremia:

1. Thirst, irritability, restlessness.

2. Severe: lethargy, seizures, coma.

3. Causes: dehydration, diabetes insipidus, osmotic diuresis, inadequate water intake (infants, elderly).

RED FLAGS

1. Na+ <120 mmol/L or >160 mmol/L.

2. Seizures, coma, altered mental status.

3. Rapidly falling or rising sodium.

4. Hypotension, shock, or severe dehydration.

5. Pediatric or elderly patients with severe derangements.

DIFFERENTIAL DIAGNOSIS

1. Hyponatremia: SIADH, CHF, cirrhosis, renal failure, thiazides, vomiting/diarrhea.

2. Hypernatremia: dehydration, DI, osmotic diuresis, burns, GI losses.

INVESTIGATIONS

1. Serum electrolytes, osmolality, glucose, creatinine, urea.

2. Urine osmolality, urine sodium.

3. Bedside glucose to exclude hyperglycemia-related pseudohyponatremia.

4. ECG if severe disturbances or symptomatic.

MANAGEMENT IN RURAL ER (WITH DRUG DOSAGES)

Hyponatremia:

1. If severe with seizures/coma:

    - 3% NaCl 100 mL IV bolus over 10 min; may repeat up to 3 times (max 300 mL) until symptoms improve.

    - Pediatrics: 3% NaCl 2 mL/kg IV bolus (max 100 mL).

2. Target: increase Na+ by 4–6 mmol/L in 24 h (do NOT exceed 8–10 mmol/L/24h).

3. Fluid restriction in SIADH.

4. Correct hypovolemia with NS boluses (500–1000 mL adults; 20 mL/kg pediatrics).

Hypernatremia:

1. Treat underlying cause (fluids, diabetes insipidus).

2. If hypovolemic: NS 500–1000 mL (20 mL/kg pediatrics) until stable, then switch to hypotonic fluids.

3. Free water replacement: D5W IV or enteral water.

4. Correction rate: decrease Na+ by max 10–12 mmol/L per 24 h to avoid cerebral edema.

Adjuncts:

1. Seizure management: Lorazepam 0.1 mg/kg IV (max 4 mg) if seizure.

2. Monitor electrolytes q2–4h in severe cases.

WHEN TO CALL A SPECIALIST / TRANSFER

1. Na+ <120 or >160.
2. Symptomatic patients with seizures, coma, or shock.
3. Unclear etiology needing advanced diagnostics.
4. Pediatric or elderly patients with severe abnormalities.
5. All cases needing hypertonic saline or complex fluid correction.

DISPOSITION

1. Discharge: mild, asymptomatic, reversible cause corrected.
2. Admit locally: moderate abnormalities requiring monitoring.
3. Transfer: severe, symptomatic, unstable, or requiring ICU-level care.

ADMISSION ORDERS (RURAL HOSPITAL)

1. Admit to monitored bed.
2. IV fluids as indicated; strict I&O.
3. Serial sodium checks q2–4h if severe.
4. Treat underlying cause (fluid restriction, hydration, etc.).
5. Seizure precautions and monitoring.

REFERENCES

1. Emergency Care BC — Hyponatremia &

Hypernatremia: https://emergencycarebc.ca/clinical_resource

2. NICE CKS — Sodium Disorders: https://cks.nice.org.uk

3. Canadian Society of Nephrology — Electrolyte Guidance (open access): https://www.csnscn.ca

4. CDC Sodium & Health Resources: https://www.cdc.gov

5. WHO Emergency & Critical Care Guidance: https://www.who.int

SECTION VII –
INFECTIOUS DISEASES

SEPSIS RECOGNITION & MANAGEMENT — RURAL ER APPROACH

OVERVIEW

Sepsis is life-threatening organ dysfunction caused by a dysregulated host response to infection. Septic shock is defined as sepsis with persistent hypotension requiring vasopressors to maintain MAP ≥65 mmHg and lactate >2 mmol/L despite adequate fluids. In rural ERs, early recognition, resuscitation, and timely transfer are essential.

CLINICAL PRESENTATION

1. Fever, chills, rigors, malaise.
2. Hypothermia in severe cases.
3. Tachycardia, tachypnea, hypotension.
4. Altered mental status.
5. Oliguria.
6. Signs of infection: pneumonia, UTI, cellulitis, meningitis, intra-abdominal infection.

RED FLAGS

1. Hypotension (SBP <90 or MAP <65).
2. Tachypnea >22/min, SpO_2 <90%.
3. Lactate ≥2 mmol/L.
4. Altered mental status.
5. Poor perfusion: mottled skin, delayed cap refill, oliguria.

DIFFERENTIAL DIAGNOSIS

1. Hypovolemic shock (hemorrhage, dehydration).
2. Cardiogenic shock (MI, arrhythmia, tamponade).
3. Obstructive shock (PE, tension pneumothorax).
4. Anaphylaxis.

INVESTIGATIONS

Bedside:
1. Vitals, SpO_2, urine output.
2. POCUS: IVC for volume status, cardiac function, lung B-lines.

Labs:
1. CBC, electrolytes, creatinine, LFTs, lactate.
2. Blood cultures ×2 before antibiotics (do not delay >45 min).
3. Urinalysis, urine culture.
4. Cultures from suspected source.
5. CXR if pneumonia suspected.

MANAGEMENT IN RURAL ER (WITH DRUG DOSAGES)

Initial resuscitation (within 1 hour):

1. Oxygen: maintain SpO_2 ≥94%.

2. IV access ×2 large bore.

3. IV fluids: NS/LR 30 mL/kg bolus within first 3 h (peds: 20 mL/kg bolus, may repeat ×2).

Antibiotics (within 1 hour):

1. Broad-spectrum, based on source:

    • - Community-acquired pneumonia: Ceftriaxone 2 g IV daily ± Azithromycin 500 mg IV daily.

    • - Urosepsis: Ceftriaxone 2 g IV daily (peds 50 mg/kg).

    • - Intra-abdominal: Ceftriaxone 2 g IV daily + Metronidazole 500 mg IV q8h.

    • - MRSA concern: add Vancomycin 15 mg/kg IV (max 2 g).

2. Pediatric: weight-based dosing (e.g., Ceftriaxone 50 mg/kg IV daily).

Vasopressors (if shock persists after fluids):

1. Norepinephrine: 2–20 mcg/min IV infusion, titrate to MAP ≥65.

2. Pediatric: 0.05–1 mcg/kg/min.

3. If unavailable: Dopamine 5–20 mcg/kg/min.

Adjuncts:

1. Acetaminophen 650–1000 mg PO/IV q6h (peds 15 mg/kg).
2. DVT prophylaxis if admitted.
3. Stress ulcer prophylaxis if intubated/critically ill.

If refractory shock:

1. Hydrocortisone 200 mg IV/day (peds 2 mg/kg IV q6h, max 50 mg/dose).

WHEN TO CALL A SPECIALIST / TRANSFER

1. All septic shock patients.
2. Patients requiring vasopressors not available locally.
3. Pediatric or elderly septic patients with instability.
4. Any patient with multi-organ dysfunction.
5. Early contact with referral center critical.

DISPOSITION

1. Discharge: NOT appropriate if sepsis suspected.
2. Admit locally: only if mild sepsis, improving, with monitoring capacity.
3. Transfer: all septic shock, unstable, or requiring ICU-level care.

ADMISSION ORDERS (RURAL HOSPITAL)

1. Admit to monitored bed.
2. IV fluids as above.
3. IV antibiotics broad-spectrum.

4. Oxygen therapy, monitor urine output.

5. Vitals q15–30min initially.

6. Prepare for transfer if unstable.

REFERENCES

1. Surviving Sepsis Campaign (open resources): https://www.sccm.org/SurvivingSepsisCampaign

2. Emergency Care BC — Sepsis & Septic Shock: https://emergencycarebc.ca/clinical_resource

3. NICE CKS — Sepsis: https://cks.nice.org.uk

4. CDC Sepsis Resources: https://www.cdc.gov/sepsis

5. WHO Emergency & Critical Care Guidance: https://www.who.int

MENINGITIS & ENCEPHALITIS (EMPIRIC ANTIBIOTICS) — RURAL ER APPROACH

OVERVIEW

Meningitis and encephalitis are life-threatening CNS infections that require urgent recognition and immediate empiric antimicrobial therapy. Delays in antibiotics increase mortality. Rural ERs should focus on early recognition, empiric treatment, supportive care, and transfer to tertiary centers for definitive management.

CLINICAL PRESENTATION

Meningitis:
1. Fever, headache, photophobia, neck stiffness.
2. Nausea/vomiting.
3. Altered mental status, seizures in severe cases.

Encephalitis:
1. Altered behavior, confusion, seizures.
2. Fever, headache.

3. Focal neurological deficits.

4. Consider HSV encephalitis in any febrile patient with new psychiatric or seizure presentation.

RED FLAGS

1. Rapidly progressive altered LOC.

2. Seizures or status epilepticus.

3. Focal neurological deficit.

4. Septic shock, purpuric rash (meningococcemia).

5. Infants: bulging fontanelle, irritability, poor feeding.

DIFFERENTIAL DIAGNOSIS

1. Intracranial hemorrhage.

2. Stroke.

3. Severe migraine.

4. Autoimmune encephalitis.

5. CNS tumor or abscess.

6. Toxic/metabolic encephalopathy.

INVESTIGATIONS

Bedside:

1. Vitals, glucose, SpO_2.

2. Neuro exam, fundoscopy (papilledema).

Labs:

1. CBC, electrolytes, creatinine, LFTs, coagulation.

2. Blood cultures ×2 before antibiotics (do not delay >45

min).

Imaging:

1. CT head if focal neurological deficit, papilledema, immunocompromised, or seizure before LP.

Lumbar puncture (if no contraindication):

1. CSF cell count, glucose, protein, Gram stain, culture, PCR (HSV, enterovirus if available).

MANAGEMENT IN RURAL ER (WITH DRUG DOSAGES)

Immediate management:

1. Airway, breathing, circulation stabilization.
2. Oxygen to maintain SpO_2 ≥94%.
3. IV fluids: NS bolus 20 mL/kg if shock.
   - Empiric antibiotics (give within 1 hour of presentation):
   - Adults (<50 years): Ceftriaxone 2 g IV q12h.
   - Adults (≥50 years or immunocompromised): Ceftriaxone 2 g IV q12h + Vancomycin 15 mg/kg IV q8–12h + Ampicillin 2 g IV q4h (for Listeria).
   - Pediatrics (>1 month): Ceftriaxone 100 mg/kg/day IV divided q12–24h (max 4 g/day) + Vancomycin 15 mg/kg IV q6h.
   - Neonates (<1 month): Ampicillin 50 mg/kg IV q6h + Cefotaxime 50 mg/kg IV q6–8h (avoid ceftriaxone

in neonates).

Encephalitis (suspected HSV):

1. Acyclovir 10 mg/kg IV q8h (peds: 20 mg/kg IV q8h) + empiric antibiotics until bacterial meningitis ruled out.

Adjuncts:

1. Dexamethasone 10 mg IV q6h × 4 days in suspected bacterial meningitis (esp. pneumococcal).
2. Seizure control: Lorazepam 0.1 mg/kg IV (max 4 mg), then phenytoin/levetiracetam if needed.

WHEN TO CALL A SPECIALIST / TRANSFER

1. All suspected meningitis or encephalitis.
2. Infants, elderly, immunocompromised patients.
3. Refractory seizures, coma, or septic shock.
4. Arrange urgent transfer to tertiary center with neurology/infectious disease support.

DISPOSITION

1. Discharge: NOT appropriate if meningitis or encephalitis suspected.
2. Admit locally: only if mild viral meningitis proven, improving, and no red flags.
3. Transfer: all suspected bacterial meningitis or encephalitis.

ADMISSION ORDERS (RURAL HOSPITAL)

1. Admit to monitored bed if awaiting transfer.

2. IV antibiotics/acyclovir as above.

3. Oxygen, IV fluids, seizure precautions.

4. Neuro checks q1h.

5. Prepare for transfer urgently.

REFERENCES

1. Emergency Care BC — Meningitis & Encephalitis: https://emergencycarebc.ca/clinical_resource

2. NICE CKS — Meningitis, Encephalitis: https://cks.nice.org.uk

3. Canadian Paediatric Society — CNS Infections: https://cps.ca

4. CDC Meningitis & Encephalitis: https://www.cdc.gov

5. WHO Meningitis Guidance: https://www.who.int

FEVER IN THE RETURNING TRAVELER (MALARIA, DENGUE, ETC.) — RURAL ER APPROACH

OVERVIEW

Fever in the returning traveler is a diagnostic challenge in rural ERs. Malaria is the most critical 'can't miss' diagnosis due to rapid progression to severe disease and death. Other important tropical infections include dengue, typhoid, chikungunya, rickettsial infections, and viral hemorrhagic fevers. A detailed travel history, exposure risks, and rapid diagnostics (if available) are essential.

CLINICAL PRESENTATION

1. Malaria: cyclical fever, chills, sweats, headache, myalgias, GI symptoms; severe malaria may cause altered LOC, seizures, anemia, jaundice, renal failure.
2. Dengue: fever, retro-orbital pain, myalgias ('breakbone fever'), rash, bleeding, thrombocytopenia, plasma leakage (shock in severe cases).

3. Typhoid: prolonged fever, abdominal pain, constipation/diarrhea, rose spots, hepatosplenomegaly.

4. Chikungunya: fever, severe arthralgia/arthritis, rash.

5. Rickettsial disease: fever, rash, eschar at bite site.

6. Viral hemorrhagic fevers (Ebola, Lassa): fever, bleeding, hypotension, multi-organ failure (rare but critical to recognize).

RED FLAGS

1. Recent travel to malaria-endemic area (esp. sub-Saharan Africa, SE Asia, South America).

2. Severe malaria signs: impaired consciousness, seizures, severe anemia, renal failure, jaundice, respiratory distress, shock.

3. Hemorrhagic manifestations, petechiae, or GI bleeding.

4. Hypotension, tachypnea, tachycardia.

5. Pregnant women, children, immunocompromised travelers.

DIFFERENTIAL DIAGNOSIS

1. Malaria (P. falciparum, P. vivax, P. ovale, P. malariae).

2. Arboviruses: Dengue, Chikungunya, Zika.

3. Enteric fever (Typhoid, Paratyphoid).

4. Rickettsial infections.

5. Viral hepatitis.

6. Acute HIV seroconversion.

7. Common infections (pneumonia, UTI, sepsis).

INVESTIGATIONS

1. Bedside: vitals, glucose, SpO_2.

2. Labs: CBC (thrombocytopenia suggests malaria/ dengue), LFTs, renal function, electrolytes.

3. Malaria rapid diagnostic test (RDT) if available, and thick/thin smear (gold standard).

4. Dengue NS1 antigen, PCR, or serology (if available).

5. Blood cultures (typhoid).

6. CXR and urine analysis for common bacterial sources.

MANAGEMENT IN RURAL ER (WITH DRUG DOSAGES)

General:

1. Stabilize ABCs, IV fluids for hypotension (20 mL/kg bolus in children; 500–1000 mL in adults, reassess frequently).

2. Oxygen if $SpO_2 < 94\%$.

3. Antipyretics: Acetaminophen 650–1000 mg PO/ IV q6h (peds 15 mg/kg q6h). Avoid NSAIDs/aspirin in suspected dengue (bleeding risk).

Malaria (empiric if strongly suspected and diagnostic delay):

1. Severe malaria: IV Artesunate 2.4 mg/kg at 0, 12, 24 h then daily (preferred, if available). Alternative: IV Quinine 10 mg/kg IV q8h over 4 h.
2. Uncomplicated malaria: Artemether–Lumefantrine (Coartem) 20/120 mg, 4 tabs PO BID ×3 days (adult dose).
3. Pediatric dosing per weight band.

Dengue:
1. Supportive only: IV fluids judiciously (avoid fluid overload in plasma leakage phase).
2. Platelet transfusion only if life-threatening bleeding.

Typhoid fever:
1. Ceftriaxone 2 g IV daily (peds 50 mg/kg daily).
2. Azithromycin 1 g PO once daily ×5–7 days for susceptible strains.

Rickettsial disease:
1. Doxycycline 100 mg PO/IV BID (peds ≥8 years: 2.2 mg/kg BID).

Encephalopathy, seizures, shock:
1. Manage per sepsis/neurological protocols; urgent transfer.

WHEN TO CALL A SPECIALIST / TRANSFER

1. Any suspected severe malaria, dengue shock syndrome, or viral hemorrhagic fever.

2. Children, pregnant women, immunocompromised patients with fever post-travel.

3. Unstable patients needing ICU-level care.

4. Notify public health if viral hemorrhagic fever suspected.

DISPOSITION

1. Discharge: mild, well-appearing patient with reassuring workup and reliable follow-up.

2. Admit locally: stable malaria, dengue, or typhoid if safe monitoring possible.

3. Transfer: severe malaria, shock, encephalitis, hemorrhagic fever, or unstable patient.

ADMISSION ORDERS (RURAL HOSPITAL)

1. Admit to monitored bed.

2. Oxygen, IV fluids, antipyretics.

3. Start empiric therapy for malaria/typhoid if suspected.

4. Serial vitals and fluid balance.

5. Prepare for urgent transfer if deterioration.

REFERENCES

1. CDC Travelers' Health — Malaria, Dengue, Typhoid: https://wwwnc.cdc.gov/travel

2. WHO Malaria Guidelines & Dengue Guidance: https://www.who.int

3. NICE CKS — Malaria, Fever in Returning Traveler:

https://cks.nice.org.uk

4. Canadian Paediatric Society — Fever in Returning Traveler: https://cps.ca

5. Emergency Care BC — Tropical & Infectious Diseases: https://emergencycarebc.ca/clinical_ resource

COMMON RURAL OUTBREAKS (INFLUENZA, GASTROENTERITIS, COVID, TB BASICS) — RURAL ER APPROACH

OVERVIEW

Rural communities are vulnerable to outbreaks of infectious diseases due to limited resources and close community contact. Common outbreaks include influenza, viral/bacterial gastroenteritis, COVID-19, and tuberculosis (TB). The rural ER must focus on early recognition, supportive management, infection control, and public health notification.

CLINICAL PRESENTATION

Influenza:
1. Fever, myalgias, headache, sore throat, cough, fatigue.
2. High-risk: elderly, infants, pregnant, immunocompromised.

Gastroenteritis:

1. Nausea, vomiting, diarrhea, abdominal cramps.
2. Risk of dehydration, especially in children/elderly.

COVID-19:
1. Fever, cough, dyspnea, anosmia, GI symptoms.
2. Severe: hypoxemia, ARDS, sepsis.

Tuberculosis:
1. Chronic cough >2 weeks, weight loss, night sweats, hemoptysis.
2. Consider in returning travelers, immunocompromised, or community clusters.

RED FLAGS

1. Influenza/COVID: respiratory distress, hypoxemia (SpO_2 <90%), altered LOC.
2. Gastroenteritis: severe dehydration, shock, bloody diarrhea.
3. TB: hemoptysis, weight loss, suspected meningitis or miliary TB.
4. Outbreaks: multiple cases presenting from same community.

DIFFERENTIAL DIAGNOSIS

1. Influenza-like illness: RSV, adenovirus, COVID-19.
2. Gastroenteritis: food poisoning, norovirus, rotavirus, bacterial causes (Salmonella, Shigella, E. coli, Campylobacter).
3. Chronic cough: COPD, asthma, lung cancer,

fungal infections.

INVESTIGATIONS

1. Influenza: rapid antigen or PCR (if available).
2. COVID-19: PCR or rapid antigen testing.
3. Gastroenteritis: usually clinical; stool cultures for severe/prolonged cases.
4. TB: sputum AFB smear, GeneXpert (if available), CXR.

MANAGEMENT IN RURAL ER (WITH DRUG DOSAGES)

Influenza:

1. Supportive care.
2. Oseltamivir 75 mg PO BID ×5 days (peds 3 mg/kg BID if <15 kg; 45 mg BID if 15–23 kg; 60 mg BID if 23–40 kg).

Gastroenteritis:

1. Rehydration mainstay.
2. ORS if mild; IV fluids (NS/LR 20 mL/kg bolus peds; 500–1000 mL adults) if severe.
3. Ondansetron 0.15 mg/kg (max 8 mg) PO/IV for vomiting.
4. Antibiotics only if severe bacterial suspected (e.g., Ciprofloxacin 500 mg PO BID ×3–5 days for traveler's diarrhea).

COVID-19:

1. Mild: home isolation, supportive.

2. Moderate/severe: Oxygen to maintain SpO_2 ≥94%.

3. Dexamethasone 6 mg PO/IV daily ×10 days if requiring oxygen.

4. Antivirals (if available per public health guidance).

5. Anticoagulation: Enoxaparin 40 mg SC daily (peds 1 mg/kg SC q12h if high risk).

Tuberculosis:

1. Isolation (airborne precautions).

2. Notify public health immediately.

3. Do not delay empiric therapy unless directed by TB specialist.

4. Standard regimen (RIPE): Rifampin, Isoniazid, Pyrazinamide, Ethambutol (initiated under specialist guidance).

WHEN TO CALL A SPECIALIST / TRANSFER

1. Severe respiratory distress (influenza, COVID).

2. Severe dehydration from gastroenteritis.

3. Suspected or confirmed TB cases (notify public health).

4. Pediatric, elderly, or immunocompromised outbreak patients.

5. Cluster of cases suggesting outbreak — notify regional health authority.

DISPOSITION

1. Discharge: mild influenza/COVID/gastroenteritis with safe home isolation/hydration.
2. Admit locally: moderate cases requiring IV fluids, oxygen, or monitoring.
3. Transfer: severe respiratory failure, ARDS, septic shock, or complications requiring ICU.

ADMISSION ORDERS (RURAL HOSPITAL)

1. Admit to monitored bed if unstable.
2. IV fluids, oxygen, monitoring.
3. Antivirals/antibiotics as appropriate.
4. Contact/droplet/airborne precautions depending on pathogen.
5. Notify public health for outbreak reporting.

REFERENCES

1. CDC — Influenza, COVID-19, Gastroenteritis, TB: https://www.cdc.gov
2. WHO — Influenza, COVID-19, TB, Gastroenteritis Outbreaks: https://www.who.int
3. NICE CKS — Influenza, Gastroenteritis, TB: https://cks.nice.org.uk
4. Canadian Paediatric Society — Viral Infections & TB: https://cps.ca
5. Emergency Care BC — Outbreak Management Resources: https://emergencycarebc.ca/clinical_resource

TUBERCULOSIS (TB) — RURAL ER BASICS

OVERVIEW

Tuberculosis (TB) is a chronic infection caused by *Mycobacterium tuberculosis*. It remains a public health issue in many rural and Indigenous communities in Canada, as well as among returning travelers from endemic regions. TB most commonly affects the lungs (pulmonary TB) but can involve any organ (extrapulmonary TB). The rural ER role is early recognition, infection control, supportive care, and urgent referral to public health and TB specialists.

CLINICAL PRESENTATION

Pulmonary TB:
1. Chronic cough >2–3 weeks (may be productive, sometimes with hemoptysis).
2. Weight loss, night sweats, fever, fatigue.
3. Chest pain, dyspnea in advanced cases.

Extrapulmonary TB:

1. Lymphadenitis, pleural effusion, pericarditis.
2. Meningitis (headache, fever, altered mental status).
3. Bone/joint TB, renal TB.
4. Disseminated (miliary TB): multi-organ involvement, sepsis-like presentation.

RED FLAGS

1. Hemoptysis.
2. Severe weight loss, cachexia.
3. Signs of TB meningitis (headache, confusion, seizures).
4. Respiratory distress.
5. Suspected miliary TB (diffuse CXR pattern, multi-organ involvement).
6. Immunocompromised patients (HIV, transplant, chronic steroids).

DIFFERENTIAL DIAGNOSIS

1. Chronic bronchitis/COPD.
2. Lung cancer.
3. Pneumonia (bacterial, fungal).
4. Sarcoidosis.
5. Other chronic infections (non-tuberculous mycobacteria).

INVESTIGATIONS

Bedside:
1. Vitals, pulse oximetry.

Labs:
1. CBC, ESR/CRP, HIV testing (if consented).

Microbiology:
1. Sputum for acid-fast bacilli (AFB) smear and culture ×3 (early morning samples best).
2. GeneXpert MTB/RIF (if available) for rapid detection and rifampin resistance.

Imaging:
1. CXR: cavitary upper lobe lesions, hilar adenopathy, miliary pattern.
2. CT chest if available for atypical presentations.

MANAGEMENT IN RURAL ER (WITH DRUG DOSAGES)

Immediate steps:
1. Place patient in airborne isolation (negative pressure room if available, N95 masks for staff).
2. Notify local public health authority immediately.
3. Collect sputum samples for AFB.
4. DO NOT start empiric TB treatment in ER unless patient is critically ill and discussed with TB specialist.

Supportive Care:

1. Oxygen for hypoxemia.

2. IV fluids for dehydration.

3. Manage complications (e.g., hemoptysis, pleural effusion).

Standard TB Regimen (started under public health/specialist guidance):

1. RIPE therapy: Rifampin, Isoniazid, Pyrazinamide, Ethambutol.

   - - Rifampin: Adults 10 mg/kg (max 600 mg) PO daily; Peds 10–20 mg/kg (max 600 mg).

   - - Isoniazid: Adults 5 mg/kg (max 300 mg) PO daily; Peds 10 mg/kg (max 300 mg).

   - - Pyrazinamide: Adults 25 mg/kg PO daily; Peds 15–30 mg/kg (max 2 g).

   - - Ethambutol: Adults 15 mg/kg PO daily; Peds 15–25 mg/kg (max 1.6 g).

Adjuncts:

1. Pyridoxine (Vitamin B6) 25–50 mg PO daily with isoniazid to prevent neuropathy.

2. Corticosteroids in TB meningitis or pericarditis (e.g., Dexamethasone 0.4 mg/kg/day IV taper).

WHEN TO CALL A SPECIALIST / TRANSFER

1. All suspected TB cases should be discussed with infectious disease/TB program.

2. Respiratory distress, massive hemoptysis, or meningitis → urgent transfer.

3. Pediatric TB cases.

4. Multidrug-resistant TB suspicion (history of prior incomplete treatment, endemic exposure).

DISPOSITION

1. Discharge: NOT appropriate for suspected pulmonary TB without specialist/public health involvement.

2. Admit locally: only if isolation feasible and in coordination with TB program.

3. Transfer: unstable, critically ill, or where rural facilities cannot ensure airborne isolation.

ADMISSION ORDERS (RURAL HOSPITAL)

1. Airborne isolation precautions.

2. Notify public health and infectious disease.

3. Collect sputum samples.

4. Supportive care (oxygen, fluids, nutrition).

5. Prepare for transfer if unstable.

REFERENCES

1. CDC — Tuberculosis Guidance: https://www.cdc.gov/tb

2. WHO — Global TB Guidelines: https://www.who.int/teams/global-tuberculosis-programme

3. NICE CKS — Tuberculosis: https://cks.nice.org.uk

4. Canadian Tuberculosis Standards (Public Health

Agency of Canada): https://www.canada.ca

5. Emergency Care BC — Tuberculosis: https://
    emergencycarebc.ca/clinical_resource

COVID-19 — RURAL ER APPROACH

OVERVIEW

COVID-19, caused by SARS-CoV-2, remains a significant infectious disease challenge in rural ERs. While most cases are mild, severe disease can progress to hypoxemia, respiratory failure, ARDS, sepsis, or multi-organ dysfunction. Rural priorities include rapid recognition, infection control, supportive care, and transfer of severe cases.

CLINICAL PRESENTATION

1. Fever, cough, sore throat, myalgias, fatigue.
2. Loss of taste/smell (anosmia).
3. Dyspnea, hypoxemia in moderate-severe cases.
4. GI symptoms (nausea, diarrhea).
5. Severe: ARDS, sepsis, thromboembolic events, multi-organ failure.

RED FLAGS

1. SpO_2 <90% on room air.
2. Respiratory distress, tachypnea.

3. Hypotension, shock.

4. Altered mental status.

5. High-risk patients: elderly, immunocompromised, pregnant, chronic conditions (diabetes, cardiac, pulmonary).

DIFFERENTIAL DIAGNOSIS

1. Influenza, RSV, adenovirus.

2. Bacterial pneumonia.

3. Pulmonary embolism.

4. Sepsis from another source.

INVESTIGATIONS

1. Nasopharyngeal swab: COVID-19 PCR or rapid antigen.

2. CBC, electrolytes, creatinine, LFTs.

3. CXR: bilateral infiltrates in pneumonia/ARDS.

4. Pulse oximetry and ABG if hypoxemic.

5. D-dimer, CRP, ferritin if severe (risk stratification).

MANAGEMENT IN RURAL ER (WITH DRUG DOSAGES)

Supportive Care:

1. Oxygen: target SpO_2 92–96% (use nasal prongs, face mask, or HFNC if available).

2. Prone positioning in hypoxemia if tolerated.

3. IV fluids cautiously — avoid overload.

Medications:

1. Acetaminophen 650–1000 mg PO/IV q6h (peds 15 mg/kg q6h) for fever.
2. Dexamethasone 6 mg PO/IV daily ×10 days (peds 0.15 mg/kg, max 6 mg).
3. Anticoagulation (if not contraindicated):
   - - Enoxaparin 40 mg SC daily prophylaxis.
   - - Peds: 1 mg/kg SC q12h if high risk.

Antivirals/targeted therapies (if available and per public health guidance):

1. Remdesivir: 200 mg IV day 1, then 100 mg IV daily ×5 days (adults).
2. Not typically available in rural ER; start if protocol allows.

Antibiotics: only if bacterial pneumonia suspected.

Escalation:

1. If worsening respiratory failure: prepare for intubation if trained and resources available.
2. Vasopressors if shock: Norepinephrine 2–20 mcg/min IV (peds 0.05–1 mcg/kg/min).

WHEN TO CALL A SPECIALIST / TRANSFER

1. SpO_2 <90% despite oxygen.
2. ARDS, sepsis, or multi-organ dysfunction.
3. Need for mechanical ventilation.
4. High-risk patients deteriorating rapidly.

5. Contact referral/ICU center early.

DISPOSITION

1. Discharge: mild, stable, safe home isolation, no red flags.
2. Admit locally: moderate disease requiring oxygen, monitoring.
3. Transfer: severe disease requiring ventilatory support or ICU.

ADMISSION ORDERS (RURAL HOSPITAL)

1. Admit to monitored/negative pressure room if possible.
2. Oxygen therapy, prone positioning.
3. Dexamethasone, anticoagulation.
4. Supportive care: fluids, antipyretics.
5. Droplet/airborne/contact precautions.
6. Notify public health.

REFERENCES

1. CDC — COVID-19 Guidance: https://www.cdc.gov/coronavirus
2. WHO — COVID-19 Clinical Management: https://www.who.int
3. NICE CKS — COVID-19: https://cks.nice.org.uk
4. Canadian Paediatric Society — COVID-19 & Children: https://cps.ca
5. Emergency Care BC — COVID-19 Resources: https://emergencycarebc.ca/clinical_resource

GASTROENTERITIS — RURAL ER APPROACH

OVERVIEW

Gastroenteritis is a common cause of ER visits in rural settings, especially in children and elderly populations. It is usually viral (norovirus, rotavirus), but may also be bacterial (Salmonella, Shigella, Campylobacter, E. coli) or parasitic (Giardia, Cryptosporidium). The major risk is dehydration, which can rapidly progress in infants, elderly, and immunocompromised patients.

CLINICAL PRESENTATION

1. Nausea, vomiting, watery diarrhea, abdominal cramps.
2. Low-grade fever (more common in viral).
3. Bloody diarrhea suggests bacterial cause (Shigella, Campylobacter, EHEC).
4. Severe dehydration: sunken eyes, dry mucous membranes, tachycardia, hypotension, lethargy.
5. Infants: decreased feeding, few wet diapers, irritability, drowsiness.

RED FLAGS

1. Severe dehydration or shock.

2. Bloody diarrhea or dysentery.

3. High fever >39°C.

4. Altered mental status, seizures.

5. Severe abdominal pain or peritonitis.

6. Infants, elderly, immunocompromised with persistent vomiting/diarrhea.

DIFFERENTIAL DIAGNOSIS

1. Viral gastroenteritis (norovirus, rotavirus).

2. Bacterial enteritis (Salmonella, Shigella, Campylobacter, EHEC).

3. Parasitic infections (Giardia, Cryptosporidium).

4. Food poisoning (Staph aureus, Bacillus cereus).

5. Appendicitis, intussusception (if severe abdominal pain, pediatric).

INVESTIGATIONS

1. Usually clinical diagnosis.

2. Labs if severe: CBC, electrolytes, creatinine.

3. Stool cultures for bloody diarrhea, persistent >7 days, outbreak situations.

4. Consider O&P (ova/parasite) if travel or chronic symptoms.

5. Rapid antigen test for rotavirus in children (if available).

MANAGEMENT IN RURAL ER (WITH DRUG DOSAGES)

Rehydration:

1. ORS (oral rehydration solution) for mild-moderate dehydration.
2. IV fluids for severe dehydration/shock:
   - - Adults: NS or LR 500–1000 mL bolus, repeat as needed.
   - - Pediatrics: 20 mL/kg NS or LR bolus, may repeat ×2.

Antiemetics:

1. Ondansetron 4–8 mg PO/IV q6–8h (peds 0.15 mg/kg, max 8 mg).
2. Metoclopramide 10 mg IV q6–8h (peds 0.1–0.15 mg/kg).

Antipyretics:

1. Acetaminophen 650–1000 mg PO/IV q6h (peds 15 mg/kg q6h).

Antibiotics (only for selected cases):

1. Ciprofloxacin 500 mg PO BID ×3–5 days (traveler's diarrhea, severe bacterial cases).
2. Azithromycin 1 g PO once or 500 mg PO daily ×3 days (Campylobacter, traveler's diarrhea).
3. Avoid antibiotics in EHEC (risk of HUS).

Adjuncts:

1. Zinc supplementation in children with diarrhea: 20 mg PO daily ×10–14 days (10 mg if <6 months).

2. Probiotics may shorten illness duration.

WHEN TO CALL A SPECIALIST / TRANSFER

1. Severe dehydration or shock not responding to fluids.

2. Persistent bloody diarrhea or suspected HUS.

3. Infants/elderly with severe electrolyte abnormalities.

4. Outbreak situations requiring public health involvement.

DISPOSITION

1. Discharge: mild cases, tolerating PO, reliable follow-up.

2. Admit locally: moderate dehydration needing IV fluids.

3. Transfer: severe dehydration, shock, suspected HUS, or critically ill.

ADMISSION ORDERS (RURAL HOSPITAL)

1. IV fluids, monitor electrolytes.

2. Antiemetics/antipyretics.

3. Stool cultures if indicated.

4. Strict I&O, recheck vitals frequently.

5. Contact precautions for infectious diarrhea.

REFERENCES

1. CDC — Viral Gastroenteritis Guidance: https://www.cdc.gov

2. WHO — Diarrhoeal Disease & ORS Protocols: https://www.who.int

3. NICE CKS — Gastroenteritis: https://cks.nice.org.uk

4. Canadian Paediatric Society — Acute Gastroenteritis in Children: https://cps.ca

5. Emergency Care BC — Gastroenteritis Management: https://emergencycarebc.ca/clinical_resource

INFLUENZA — RURAL ER APPROACH

OVERVIEW

Influenza is an acute viral respiratory illness that occurs seasonally and can spread rapidly in rural communities with limited healthcare resources. Most cases are self-limited, but severe illness can occur in high-risk groups (infants, elderly, pregnant, immunocompromised, chronic disease). Rural ER priorities are early recognition, supportive care, antiviral therapy for eligible patients, and outbreak prevention.

CLINICAL PRESENTATION

1. Sudden onset fever, chills, malaise, myalgias.
2. Cough, sore throat, rhinorrhea.
3. Headache, fatigue, anorexia.
4. Children may present with GI symptoms (vomiting, diarrhea).
5. Severe: pneumonia, hypoxemia, sepsis, encephalopathy.

RED FLAGS

1. Hypoxemia (SpO_2 <90%).
2. Respiratory distress, tachypnea, retractions (pediatrics).
3. Altered mental status.
4. Severe dehydration.
5. High-risk groups: <5 years, >65 years, pregnant/postpartum, chronic cardiac/respiratory disease, immunosuppression, First Nations communities (higher severity risk).

DIFFERENTIAL DIAGNOSIS

1. Other viral respiratory infections (RSV, adenovirus, COVID-19).
2. Bacterial pneumonia.
3. Sepsis.
4. Asthma/COPD exacerbation.

INVESTIGATIONS

1. Usually clinical diagnosis in season.
2. Influenza rapid antigen or PCR if available (not required for routine management).
3. CXR if concern for pneumonia.
4. CBC, electrolytes, renal/liver function in severe cases.

MANAGEMENT IN RURAL ER (WITH DRUG DOSAGES)

Supportive Care:

1. Oxygen to maintain SpO_2 ≥94%.
2. IV fluids for dehydration: NS/LR bolus 500–1000 mL adults; 20 mL/kg pediatrics.
3. Antipyretics: Acetaminophen 650–1000 mg PO/IV q6h (peds 15 mg/kg q6h, max 75 mg/kg/day).
4. Avoid aspirin in children (risk of Reye syndrome).

Antivirals (best within 48 h of onset or any severe/high-risk patient):

1. Oseltamivir (Tamiflu):
   - - Adults: 75 mg PO BID × 5 days.
   - - Pediatrics: <15 kg: 30 mg PO BID × 5 days; 15–23 kg: 45 mg PO BID × 5 days; 23–40 kg: 60 mg PO BID × 5 days; >40 kg: 75 mg PO BID × 5 days.
2. Immunocompromised/severe cases: may require 10-day course.
3. Zanamivir (inhaled): 10 mg (2 inhalations) BID × 5 days (not for <7 years).

Antibiotics: Only if bacterial pneumonia suspected (e.g., Ceftriaxone 2 g IV daily or Amoxicillin 1 g PO TID).

WHEN TO CALL A SPECIALIST / TRANSFER

1. Severe respiratory distress, hypoxemia not improved

with oxygen.

2. Altered mental status, seizures, or sepsis.

3. Infants, elderly, pregnant women with severe illness.

4. Outbreak management requiring public health coordination.

DISPOSITION

1. Discharge: Mild illness, stable, tolerating PO, reliable follow-up.

2. Admit locally: Moderate disease needing IV fluids or oxygen.

3. Transfer: Severe illness requiring advanced airway, ventilation, or ICU care.

ADMISSION ORDERS (RURAL HOSPITAL)

1. Admit to monitored bed.

2. Oxygen as needed.

3. IV fluids, antipyretics.

4. Oseltamivir as per dosing above.

5. Droplet/contact precautions.

6. Monitor vitals and urine output.

REFERENCES

1. CDC — Influenza Guidance: https://www.cdc.gov/flu

2. WHO — Influenza Fact Sheet & Guidelines: https://www.who.int

3. NICE CKS — Influenza: https://cks.nice.org.uk

4. Canadian Paediatric Society — Antiviral Use in Influenza: https://cps.ca

5. Emergency Care BC — Influenza Management: https://emergencycarebc.ca/clinical_resource

SKIN & SOFT TISSUE INFECTIONS (CELLULITIS, ERYSIPELAS, ABSCESS, MRSA, NECROTIZING FASCIITIS) — RURAL ER APPROACH

OVERVIEW

Skin and soft tissue infections (SSTIs) range from mild cellulitis to life-threatening necrotizing fasciitis.

- - Cellulitis: infection of dermis/subcutaneous tissue, poorly demarcated.
- - Erysipelas: superficial cellulitis with raised, sharply demarcated margins (Group A Strep).
- - Abscess: localized pus collection, usually requires drainage.
- - MRSA (community-acquired): increasing prevalence; consider in purulent infections.
- - Necrotizing fasciitis: rapidly progressive, life-threatening infection requiring emergent surgery.

CLINICAL PRESENTATION

1. Cellulitis: erythema, warmth, edema, tenderness, ill-defined borders.

2. Erysipelas: bright red, raised, well-demarcated lesion, fever, often face/legs.

3. Abscess: fluctuant, tender mass ± drainage.

4. MRSA: purulent SSTIs, boils, abscesses, non-response to β-lactams.

5. Necrotizing Fasciitis: severe pain out of proportion, rapidly spreading erythema, bullae, skin necrosis, crepitus, systemic toxicity.

RED FLAGS

1. Hypotension, tachycardia, systemic toxicity.

2. Rapid progression of erythema/swelling.

3. Pain out of proportion to exam.

4. Skin necrosis, bullae, crepitus.

5. Failure to improve on oral antibiotics.

DIFFERENTIAL DIAGNOSIS

1. DVT (leg swelling/redness).

2. Contact dermatitis.

3. Venous stasis dermatitis.

4. Gout, pseudogout.

5. Insect bite/allergic reaction.

INVESTIGATIONS

1. Clinical diagnosis mostly.
2. CBC, CRP, lactate if systemic toxicity.
3. Blood cultures if febrile, immunocompromised, or severe.
4. Swab/pus culture for abscess/MRSA.
5. Ultrasound for abscess vs cellulitis; CT/MRI if nec fasc suspected.

MANAGEMENT IN RURAL ER (WITH DRUG DOSAGES)

General:
1. Elevate limb, analgesia, mark borders, reassess.

Analgesia:
1. Acetaminophen 15 mg/kg PO q6h (max 1 g).
2. Ibuprofen 10 mg/kg q6–8h.
3. Morphine 0.1 mg/kg IV if severe.

Antibiotics:

Mild cellulitis/erysipelas (oral, outpatient if stable):
1. Cephalexin 500 mg PO QID (peds 25 mg/kg/dose PO q6h, max 500 mg).
2. OR Amoxicillin 500 mg PO TID.

Moderate/severe cellulitis (IV, admit):
1. Cefazolin 2 g IV q8h (peds 50 mg/kg IV q8h).

2. If penicillin allergy: Clindamycin 600 mg IV q8h (peds 10 mg/kg q8h).

MRSA suspected (purulent, abscess, treatment failure):

1. TMP-SMX 1 DS tab PO BID (peds 4–6 mg/kg TMP PO q12h).
2. OR Doxycycline 100 mg PO BID (>8 yrs).
3. OR Vancomycin 15 mg/kg IV q8–12h (max 2 g/ dose).

Abscess:

1. Incision & drainage (I&D) is primary therapy.
2. Antibiotics if systemic illness, multiple lesions, immunocompromised, extremes of age, or poor response to drainage.

Necrotizing Fasciitis:

1. Immediate surgical consultation + urgent transfer.
2. Broad-spectrum empiric: Piperacillin-Tazobactam 4.5 g IV q6h + Clindamycin 900 mg IV q8h ± Vancomycin.

WHEN TO CALL A SPECIALIST / TRANSFER

1. Necrotizing fasciitis suspected.
2. Severe systemic toxicity, sepsis.
3. Rapid progression despite antibiotics.
4. Immunocompromised patient.
5. Large/deep abscess not drainable locally.

DISPOSITION

1. Discharge: mild cellulitis/erysipelas, stable, reliable follow-up.
2. Admit locally: moderate/severe cellulitis requiring IV antibiotics.
3. Transfer: necrotizing fasciitis, unstable patients, surgical I&D beyond local capacity.

ADMISSION ORDERS (RURAL HOSPITAL)

1. Admit to monitored bed if systemic signs.
2. IV antibiotics as above.
3. Strict limb elevation.
4. Mark margins, reassess q6–8h.
5. NPO if nec fasc suspected (surgery).

REFERENCES

1. Emergency Care BC — Cellulitis, Abscess, Necrotizing Fasciitis: https://emergencycarebc.ca/clinical_resource
2. NICE CKS — Cellulitis, Skin Infections: https://cks.nice.org.uk
3. CDC — MRSA & Skin Infections Guidelines: https://www.cdc.gov
4. WHO — Antimicrobial Stewardship & SSTI Care: https://www.who.int
5. Canadian Paediatric Society — SSTIs in Children: https://cps.ca

SECTION VIII –
ONCOLOGIC EMERGENCIES

ONCOLOGIC EMERGENCIES — RURAL ER APPROACH

OVERVIEW

Oncologic emergencies are acute, potentially life-threatening complications of cancer or its treatment. Rural ER physicians must promptly recognize and stabilize these conditions while arranging transfer for definitive oncology care. Key emergencies include spinal cord compression, superior vena cava (SVC) syndrome, tumor lysis syndrome, hypercalcemia of malignancy, febrile neutropenia, and massive hemorrhage.

CLINICAL PRESENTATION

Spinal cord compression:
1. Back pain, weakness, sensory changes, incontinence.

SVC syndrome:
1. Facial/upper extremity swelling, dyspnea, cough, distended neck veins.

Tumor lysis syndrome:

1. Nausea, vomiting, diarrhea, arrhythmias, seizures.
2. Electrolyte abnormalities ($\uparrow$K+, $\uparrow$phosphate, $\downarrow$Ca2+, $\uparrow$uric acid).

Hypercalcemia of malignancy:

1. Polyuria, polydipsia, confusion, constipation, arrhythmias.

Febrile neutropenia:

1. Fever $\geq$38.0°C, neutrophils <500/μL.
2. Minimal signs of infection due to immunosuppression.

Massive hemorrhage:

1. Hemoptysis, GI bleed, tumor-related bleeding.

RED FLAGS

1. Rapid neurological deterioration (cord compression).
2. Airway compromise or severe dyspnea (SVC syndrome).
3. Seizures, arrhythmias (tumor lysis, hypercalcemia).
4. Fever with neutropenia (risk of overwhelming sepsis).
5. Uncontrolled bleeding or shock.

DIFFERENTIAL DIAGNOSIS

1. Non-oncologic causes of shock (sepsis, trauma, hemorrhage).

2. Pulmonary embolism vs. SVC syndrome.

3. Metabolic encephalopathy vs. brain metastases.

4. Other causes of back pain/neurologic deficits (disc herniation, abscess).

INVESTIGATIONS

Bedside:

1. Vitals, pulse oximetry, ECG, urine output.

Labs:

1. CBC, electrolytes, calcium, phosphate, uric acid, renal function, coagulation.

2. Blood cultures in febrile neutropenia.

Imaging:

1. MRI spine for cord compression (if available).

2. CXR/CT chest for SVC syndrome.

3. Ultrasound/CT abdomen for obstructive uropathy or bleeding source.

MANAGEMENT IN RURAL ER (WITH DRUG DOSAGES)

Spinal Cord Compression:

1. Dexamethasone 10 mg IV bolus, then 4 mg IV q6h.

2. Analgesia: Morphine 2–5 mg IV q2–4h PRN.

3. Urgent oncology/neurosurgery referral.

SVC Syndrome:

1. Elevate head of bed, oxygen.

2. Dexamethasone 10 mg IV bolus.

3. Avoid diuretics unless fluid overload.

4. Transfer for oncology/radiotherapy.

Tumor Lysis Syndrome:

1. Aggressive IV hydration: NS 200–300 mL/hr (peds 3 L/ m^2/day).

2. Allopurinol 300 mg PO daily (peds 10 mg/kg/day divided TID).

3. Rasburicase 0.2 mg/kg IV once (if available).

4. Correct electrolytes, monitor K+, phosphate, Ca2+.

Hypercalcemia of Malignancy:

1. IV NS 1–2 L bolus, then 150–200 mL/hr.

2. Calcitonin 4 IU/kg SC/IM q12h.

3. Bisphosphonates (if available): Zoledronic acid 4 mg IV over 15 min or Pamidronate 90 mg IV over 2–4 h.

Febrile Neutropenia:

1. Start antibiotics within 1 hour: Piperacillin–Tazobactam 4.5 g IV q6h (peds 80 mg/kg IV q6h, max 4.5 g/dose).

2. Alternatives: Cefepime 2 g IV q8h (peds 50 mg/kg q8h).

3. Vancomycin 15 mg/kg IV q12h if MRSA suspected.

Massive Hemorrhage:

1. ABCs, large-bore IV access.
2. Blood products: PRBCs, FFP, platelets as available.
3. Tranexamic acid: 1 g IV over 10 min, then 1 g IV over 8 h (peds 15 mg/kg, max 1 g/dose).
4. Direct pressure, packing, topical hemostatics.
5. Consult surgery/interventional radiology.

WHEN TO CALL A SPECIALIST / TRANSFER

1. Any suspected cord compression or SVC syndrome.
2. Severe TLS, refractory hypercalcemia.
3. Febrile neutropenia with sepsis.
4. Uncontrolled hemorrhage.
5. All cases requiring oncology input.

DISPOSITION

1. Discharge: not appropriate for most oncologic emergencies.
2. Admit locally: if mild hypercalcemia or febrile neutropenia stable, with oncology guidance.
3. Transfer: most cases (cord compression, SVC syndrome, TLS, unstable patients).

ADMISSION ORDERS (RURAL HOSPITAL)

1. Admit to monitored bed.
2. IV fluids, oxygen, telemetry.
3. Dexamethasone for cord compression/SVC.
4. Empiric antibiotics for neutropenia.

5. Electrolyte monitoring q4–6h.

6. Notify oncology and public health if outbreak-related.

REFERENCES

1. Emergency Care BC — Oncologic Emergencies: https://emergencycarebc.ca/clinical_resource

2. NICE CKS — Malignancy-related Emergencies: https://cks.nice.org.uk

3. CDC Cancer & Emergency Complications Resources: https://www.cdc.gov

4. WHO Palliative and Cancer Emergency Care Guidance: https://www.who.int

5. Canadian Cancer Society — Emergency Complications of Cancer: https://cancer.ca

SPINAL CORD COMPRESSION — RURAL ER APPROACH

OVERVIEW

Malignant spinal cord compression (MSCC) occurs when tumor mass, usually from vertebral metastasis, compresses the spinal cord or cauda equina. It is a time-sensitive oncologic emergency requiring immediate recognition and intervention to prevent irreversible paralysis. Most commonly associated cancers: breast, prostate, lung, renal, thyroid, lymphoma, and myeloma. Thoracic spine is most often affected (70%), followed by lumbar (20%) and cervical (10%). Rural ER priorities include rapid recognition, immediate corticosteroids, pain control, immobilization, and urgent transfer to oncology or neurosurgery.

CLINICAL PRESENTATION

1. Persistent, progressive back pain, worse at night or when lying flat.
2. Radicular pain (shooting pain radiating along a

dermatome).

3. Motor weakness (legs > arms if thoracic/lumbar).

4. Sensory loss, paresthesias.

5. Autonomic dysfunction: urinary retention, incontinence, constipation.

6. Late findings: paraplegia, quadriplegia.

RED FLAGS

1. New or worsening motor weakness.

2. Bowel/bladder dysfunction.

3. Saddle anesthesia.

4. Rapid progression of neurologic deficits.

5. Known cancer patient with new severe back pain.

DIFFERENTIAL DIAGNOSIS

1. Disc herniation.

2. Spinal abscess (epidural abscess).

3. Vertebral fracture (traumatic or pathologic).

4. Transverse myelitis.

5. Guillain–Barré syndrome (if ascending paralysis).

INVESTIGATIONS

Bedside:

1. Vitals, neurological exam.

Imaging:

1. MRI spine (whole spine if available) is the gold

standard.

2. CT myelogram if MRI unavailable.

Labs:

1. CBC, electrolytes, renal/liver function.
2. ESR/CRP if infection a concern.

MANAGEMENT IN RURAL ER (WITH DRUG DOSAGES)

Immediate measures:

1. Keep patient on strict bed rest, spinal precautions.
2. High-dose corticosteroids: Dexamethasone 10 mg IV bolus, then 4 mg IV q6h. (Pediatrics: 0.25–0.5 mg/kg IV bolus, max 10 mg; then 0.25 mg/kg q6h).
3. Analgesia: Morphine 2–5 mg IV q2–4h PRN (peds 0.05–0.1 mg/kg).
4. NSAIDs as adjunct if not contraindicated.

Supportive:

1. IV fluids as needed.
2. Bladder catheterization if retention.
3. Bowel regimen for constipation.

Definitive management requires oncology/neurosurgery (radiotherapy or decompressive surgery).

WHEN TO CALL A SPECIALIST / TRANSFER

1. All suspected cases of MSCC require urgent transfer.

2. Consult oncology/neurosurgery immediately.

3. Early transfer improves functional outcomes significantly.

DISPOSITION

1. Discharge: never appropriate.

2. Admit locally only if awaiting transfer and patient stable.

3. Transfer urgently to center with neurosurgical/ oncology capacity.

ADMISSION ORDERS (RURAL HOSPITAL)

1. Bed rest with spine precautions.

2. Dexamethasone IV as above.

3. Analgesia.

4. Foley catheter if urinary retention.

5. Monitor neuro status q2–4h.

6. Prepare transfer documentation and imaging.

REFERENCES

1. Emergency Care BC — Malignant Spinal Cord Compression: https://emergencycarebc.ca/clinical_ resource

2. NICE CKS — Spinal Cord Compression: https://cks. nice.org.uk

3. Canadian Cancer Society — Spinal Cord Compression: https://cancer.ca

4. CDC Cancer Complications Resources: https://

www.cdc.gov

5. WHO Cancer Emergency Guidance: https://www.who.int

SUPERIOR VENA CAVA (SVC) SYNDROME — RURAL ER APPROACH

OVERVIEW

Superior Vena Cava (SVC) Syndrome occurs when blood flow through the superior vena cava is obstructed, usually due to malignancy (lung cancer, lymphoma, metastatic tumors). It presents with facial and upper extremity swelling, venous congestion, and can progress to airway compromise or cerebral edema. SVC syndrome is an oncologic emergency; rural ER management focuses on stabilization, corticosteroids, oxygen, and urgent transfer.

CLINICAL PRESENTATION

1. Facial, neck, and upper extremity swelling.
2. Dyspnea, cough, orthopnea.
3. Distended neck/chest wall veins.
4. Headache, dizziness, syncope ($\uparrow$ intracranial pressure).
5. Stridor, hoarseness if airway involvement.

6. Severe: confusion, obtundation from cerebral edema.

RED FLAGS

1. Stridor or impending airway obstruction.
2. Severe dyspnea, hypoxemia.
3. Neurological deficits, altered LOC.
4. Rapid symptom progression.

DIFFERENTIAL DIAGNOSIS

1. Pericardial tamponade.
2. Pulmonary embolism.
3. Heart failure with elevated venous pressure.
4. Mediastinitis or goiter compressing great vessels.

INVESTIGATIONS

Bedside:

1. Vitals, O_2 saturation.

Imaging:

1. CXR: widened mediastinum, right upper lobe mass, pleural effusion.
2. CT chest with contrast (if available) for diagnosis and planning.

Labs:

1. CBC, electrolytes, renal/liver function.
2. Coagulation profile.

3. Blood cultures if fever (exclude infection).

MANAGEMENT IN RURAL ER (WITH DRUG DOSAGES)

Stabilization:

1. Elevate head of bed to 30–45° to reduce venous pressure.
2. Oxygen to maintain SpO_2 ≥94%.
3. IV access in lower extremities (upper limb lines may worsen obstruction).

Medications:

1. Dexamethasone 10 mg IV bolus, then 4 mg IV q6h (peds 0.25–0.5 mg/kg, max 10 mg bolus).
2. Analgesia: Morphine 2–5 mg IV q2–4h PRN (peds 0.05–0.1 mg/kg).
3. Diuretics (if severe venous congestion/edema): Furosemide 20–40 mg IV (peds 1 mg/kg, max 20 mg).

If concern for thrombus (SVC thrombosis):

1. Anticoagulation: Enoxaparin 1 mg/kg SC q12h (peds 1 mg/kg SC q12h).
2. Avoid until discussed with oncology/hematology if bleeding risk high.

Definitive management (specialist care):

1. Radiotherapy for chemosensitive tumors (lymphoma, SCLC).

2. Chemotherapy (lymphoma, germ cell tumors).

3. Endovascular stenting (preferred if available).

WHEN TO CALL A SPECIALIST / TRANSFER

1. All suspected SVC syndrome should be discussed with oncology.

2. Immediate transfer if airway compromise, cerebral edema, or hemodynamic instability.

3. Coordinate with referral center for radiotherapy, stenting, or chemotherapy.

DISPOSITION

1. Discharge: not appropriate.

2. Admit locally if awaiting transfer and stable.

3. Transfer urgently if airway compromise, severe hypoxemia, or neurological decline.

ADMISSION ORDERS (RURAL HOSPITAL)

1. Admit to monitored bed with head of bed elevated.

2. Oxygen therapy.

3. IV Dexamethasone as above.

4. Lower extremity IV access.

5. Foley catheter if significant edema.

6. Prepare documentation and imaging for transfer.

REFERENCES

1. Emergency Care BC — Superior Vena Cava

Syndrome: https://emergencycarebc.ca/clinical_
resource

2. NICE CKS — SVC Obstruction: https://cks.nice.org.uk

3. Canadian Cancer Society — SVC Syndrome:
https://cancer.ca

4. CDC Cancer-Related Complications: https://www.
cdc.gov

5. WHO Cancer Emergency Guidance: https://www.
who.int

FEBRILE NEUTROPENIA — RURAL ER APPROACH

OVERVIEW

Febrile neutropenia is defined as a single oral temperature ≥38.0°C (100.4°F) with an absolute neutrophil count (ANC) <500/μL, or expected to fall below 500/μL within 48 hours. It is a life-threatening oncologic emergency due to the high risk of overwhelming sepsis with minimal clinical signs. Rural ER priorities include rapid recognition, immediate empiric broad-spectrum antibiotics (within 1 hour), hemodynamic stabilization, and urgent coordination with oncology/infectious diseases.

CLINICAL PRESENTATION

1. Fever may be the only symptom.
2. Chills, rigors, malaise, hypotension.
3. Subtle or absent localizing signs of infection.
4. Possible mucositis, cough, dysuria, abdominal pain.

5. Severe cases: septic shock, altered LOC, multi-organ failure.

RED FLAGS

1. Hypotension (SBP <90 mmHg).
2. Tachypnea, SpO_2 <90%.
3. Altered mental status.
4. Neutrophil count <100/μL.
5. Rapid clinical deterioration despite fluids.
6. Pediatric or elderly patient with comorbidities.

DIFFERENTIAL DIAGNOSIS

1. Sepsis from any source (respiratory, urinary, GI, skin/line infection).
2. Viral infections (HSV, VZV, influenza).
3. Fungal infections (Candida, Aspergillus).
4. Non-infectious: drug fever, transfusion reaction, tumor fever.

INVESTIGATIONS

Bedside:
1. Vitals, SpO_2, urine output.

Labs:
1. CBC with differential, renal/liver function, electrolytes.
2. Lactate, CRP, procalcitonin (if available).
3. Blood cultures ×2 (from peripheral and central line

if present).

4. Urine analysis and culture.

5. Sputum culture, wound/line cultures if indicated.

Imaging:

1. CXR for cough, dyspnea, hypoxemia.

2. Consider CT chest/abdomen in persistent fever (at referral center).

MANAGEMENT IN RURAL ER (WITH DRUG DOSAGES)

Immediate empiric antibiotics (within 1 hour of triage):

1. Piperacillin–Tazobactam 4.5 g IV q6h (peds 80 mg/kg IV q6h, max 4.5 g/dose).

2. OR Cefepime 2 g IV q8h (peds 50 mg/kg IV q8h).

3. If MRSA suspected (line infection, skin/soft tissue, pneumonia): add Vancomycin 15 mg/kg IV q8–12h (max 2 g/dose).

4. If unstable/septic shock: consider dual coverage (Pip-Tazo + Vancomycin + Aminoglycoside [Gentamicin 5–7 mg/kg IV once]).

Adjunctive measures:

1. Oxygen, IV fluids: NS bolus 500–1000 mL adults (20 mL/kg peds), reassess frequently.

2. Acetaminophen 650–1000 mg PO/IV q6h (peds 15 mg/kg q6h).

3. Avoid NSAIDs/rectal meds (risk of bleeding,

mucositis).

Growth factors:

1. G-CSF (Filgrastim) 5 mcg/kg SC daily may be considered if profound neutropenia and expected prolonged recovery, but initiate in consultation with oncology.

WHEN TO CALL A SPECIALIST / TRANSFER

1. All febrile neutropenia cases require oncology/ infectious disease input.
2. Immediate transfer if unstable, septic shock, or no ICU capacity locally.
3. Pediatric febrile neutropenia requires urgent transfer.
4. Consider local admission if stable, low-risk, and antibiotics available.

DISPOSITION

1. Discharge: not appropriate.
2. Admit locally: stable, low-risk patients if oncology consulted and monitoring available.
3. Transfer: unstable, septic shock, pediatric, or no oncology support.

ADMISSION ORDERS (RURAL HOSPITAL)

1. Admit to monitored bed.
2. IV broad-spectrum antibiotics as above.

3. IV fluids, oxygen, antipyretics.

4. Strict I&O, monitor urine output.

5. Daily CBC, electrolytes, renal function.

6. Isolation precautions (neutropenic precautions).

REFERENCES

1. Emergency Care BC — Febrile Neutropenia: https://emergencycarebc.ca/clinical_resource

2. NICE CKS — Neutropenic Sepsis: https://cks.nice.org.uk

3. Canadian Cancer Society — Febrile Neutropenia: https://cancer.ca

4. CDC — Cancer & Infection Risk: https://www.cdc.gov

5. WHO — Infection Prevention in Cancer Patients: https://www.who.int

SECTION IX –
TRAUMA AND ORTHOPEDIC

COMMON FRACTURES & DISLOCATIONS (INITIAL SPLINTING, TRANSFER CRITERIA) — RURAL ER APPROACH

OVERVIEW

Fractures and dislocations are common presentations in rural ER practice. Priorities include early recognition, pain management, immobilization, and ruling out neurovascular compromise. In rural settings, temporary splinting and stabilization are often performed before definitive orthopedic management at referral centers.

CLINICAL PRESENTATION

1. Pain, swelling, deformity at the site.
2. Loss of function or range of motion.
3. Crepitus or instability.
4. Neurovascular changes: numbness, weakness, absent pulses (orthopedic emergency).

RED FLAGS

1. Absent distal pulses.
2. Severe pain out of proportion (consider compartment syndrome).
3. Open fractures.
4. Associated neuro deficit.
5. Fracture-dislocation (hip, knee, elbow).

DIFFERENTIAL DIAGNOSIS

1. Sprain or strain.
2. Ligament tear.
3. Tendon rupture.
4. Septic joint (if swelling + fever).

INVESTIGATIONS

1. X-rays: AP and lateral views including the joint above and below.
2. Bedside Doppler if pulses not palpable.
3. CBC, coagulation, type and cross if surgical transfer anticipated.

MANAGEMENT IN RURAL ER (WITH DRUG DOSAGES)

General principles:
1. Immobilize first, analgesia early.
2. Check neurovascular status before and after

immobilization.

3. Avoid repeated attempts at reduction unless critical.

Analgesia/Sedation:

1. Acetaminophen 15 mg/kg PO/IV q6h (max 1 g).
2. Ibuprofen 10 mg/kg PO q6–8h (if >6 months).
3. Morphine 0.1 mg/kg IV q2–4h (max 5 mg/dose).
4. Procedural sedation (if reduction required):
   - - Ketamine 1–2 mg/kg IV OR 4–5 mg/kg IM.
   - - Midazolam 0.05–0.1 mg/kg IV (max 2 mg).

Initial Splinting Examples:

1. Distal radius fracture → volar slab or sugar-tong splint.
2. Ankle fracture → posterior slab with stirrup splint.
3. Elbow dislocation → posterior long arm splint at 90°.
4. Femur fracture (child) → traction splint if trained and available.

Open fractures:

1. IV antibiotics within 1 hour: Cefazolin 2 g IV q8h (peds 30 mg/kg, max 2 g).
2. Tetanus prophylaxis as indicated.
3. Sterile dressing, avoid wound probing.

WHEN TO CALL A SPECIALIST / TRANSFER

Open fractures.

1. Absent distal pulses, ischemia.

2. Compartment syndrome.

3. Intra-articular fractures.

4. Complex dislocations (hip, knee, elbow).

5. Pediatric physeal fractures requiring reduction.

DISPOSITION

1. Discharge: stable, simple fracture with proper immobilization, good NV exam, reliable follow-up.

2. Admit locally: if pain poorly controlled, comorbidities, or awaiting transfer.

3. Transfer: open/complex fractures, neurovascular injury, need for operative fixation.

ADMISSION ORDERS (RURAL HOSPITAL)

1. Splint applied, NV checks q1–2h.

2. Elevate limb, ice packs.

3. Analgesia as above.

4. IV antibiotics for open fractures.

5. NPO if transfer for surgery.

REFERENCES

1. Emergency Care BC — Orthopedic Injuries & Splinting: https://emergencycarebc.ca/clinical_resource

2. NICE CKS — Fractures & Dislocations: https://cks.nice.org.uk

3. WHO — Essential Trauma Care Guidelines: https://www.who.int

4. CDC — Injury Prevention Resources: https://www.cdc.gov

5. Canadian Paediatric Society — Pediatric Fracture Care: https://cps.ca

COMPARTMENT SYNDROME (RECOGNITION & ACTION) — RURAL ER APPROACH

OVERVIEW

Compartment syndrome is a surgical emergency caused by elevated pressure within a closed muscle compartment, leading to ischemia and necrosis. It most commonly follows fractures (tibia, forearm), crush injuries, reperfusion after ischemia, or tight casts/bandages. In rural ER, the priorities are rapid recognition, analgesia, removal of constrictive dressings, limb positioning, urgent surgical consultation, and transfer.

CLINICAL PRESENTATION

1. Pain out of proportion to injury (earliest sign).
2. Pain with passive stretch of muscles in the compartment.
3. Paresthesias, numbness.
4. Paralysis, pallor, pulselessness (late findings, not

reliable early).

5. Tense, firm compartments on palpation.

RED FLAGS

1. Severe pain unrelieved by opioids.

2. Progressive neurologic deficit (numbness, weakness).

3. Increasing analgesia requirement.

4. Delayed capillary refill despite palpable pulses.

DIFFERENTIAL DIAGNOSIS

1. Peripheral nerve injury.

2. Arterial occlusion/embolism.

3. Deep vein thrombosis.

4. Severe cellulitis.

INVESTIGATIONS

1. Clinical diagnosis — do not delay for tests.

2. Compartment pressure measurement (>30 mmHg or ΔP <30 mmHg) if available, but do not wait if strong suspicion.

3. Basic labs: CBC, electrolytes, CK, creatinine (for rhabdomyolysis).

MANAGEMENT IN RURAL ER (WITH DRUG DOSAGES)

Immediate Actions:

1. Remove dressings, casts, or splints.

2. Keep limb at heart level (not elevated, not dependent).

3. Oxygen, IV fluids (NS/LR bolus 20 mL/kg if shock).

4. Foley catheter for urine monitoring.

Analgesia:

1. Morphine 0.1 mg/kg IV q2–4h (max 5 mg).

2. Ketamine 1–2 mg/kg IV for procedural pain if reduction attempted.

3. Avoid regional blocks (mask symptoms).

Antibiotics (if open fracture):

1. Cefazolin 2 g IV q8h (peds 30 mg/kg, max 2 g).

2. Add Gentamicin 5 mg/kg IV for grossly contaminated wounds.

Definitive management:

1. Emergent fasciotomy required — not typically done in rural ER unless trained and no transfer possible.

2. Urgent transfer to orthopedic/trauma center.

WHEN TO CALL A SPECIALIST / TRANSFER

1. Any suspected compartment syndrome.

2. Worsening neurovascular status.

3. Open fracture with tense compartments.

4. Delay to OR >6 hours → risk of permanent disability.

DISPOSITION

1. Never discharge suspected cases.

2. Transfer urgently for fasciotomy.

3. Admit only if awaiting immediate transfer.

ADMISSION ORDERS (RURAL HOSPITAL)

1. Strict limb monitoring q15–30 min.

2. IV fluids, analgesia.

3. NPO for possible surgery.

4. Prepare for urgent transfer.

5. Document serial neurovascular exams.

REFERENCES

1. Emergency Care BC — Compartment Syndrome: https://emergencycarebc.ca/clinical_resource

2. NICE CKS — Orthopedic Emergencies: https://cks.nice.org.uk

3. WHO — Essential Trauma Care Guidelines: https://www.who.int

4. CDC — Injury & Trauma Emergency Care: https://www.cdc.gov

5. Canadian Orthopaedic Association — Open Access Statements: https://coa-aco.org

WOUND MANAGEMENT (CLOSURE, TETANUS, ANTIBIOTICS FOR BITES/OPEN WOUNDS) — RURAL ER APPROACH

OVERVIEW

Wound management is a frequent presentation in rural ERs. Principles include hemostasis, irrigation, debridement, closure when appropriate, tetanus prophylaxis, and antibiotics for high-risk wounds. Rural priorities include safe closure of clean wounds, avoidance of infection in contaminated wounds, and timely referral when surgical repair is required.

CLINICAL PRESENTATION

1. Simple lacerations: bleeding, pain, visible wound.
2. Contaminated wounds: dirt, debris, crush mechanism.
3. Bite wounds: puncture marks, tearing, risk of polymicrobial infection.
4. Open fractures or tendon injuries: exposed bone, loss of function.

RED FLAGS

1. Gross contamination (farm injury, fecal contamination).
2. Open fracture.
3. Neurovascular compromise.
4. Deep puncture wounds (cat bites, clenched fist injuries).
5. Suspected retained foreign body.
6. Delayed presentation (>12 hours for extremity, >24 hours for face/scalp).

DIFFERENTIAL DIAGNOSIS

1. Simple laceration.
2. Complex wound (crush, avulsion).
3. Puncture wound or bite.
4. Open fracture.
5. Skin/soft tissue infection or necrotizing fasciitis (late complication).

INVESTIGATIONS

1. Clinical diagnosis, wound exploration.
2. X-ray if concern for foreign body or fracture.
3. CBC, cultures if wound infected.
4. Consider ultrasound for radiolucent FB (wood, plastic).

MANAGEMENT IN RURAL ER (WITH DRUG DOSAGES)

General principles:

1. Analgesia: Acetaminophen 15 mg/kg q6h, Ibuprofen 10 mg/kg q6–8h, Morphine 0.1 mg/kg IV if severe.

2. Local anesthesia: Lidocaine 1% without epi (max 4.5 mg/kg), with epi (max 7 mg/kg). Avoid epi in fingers, toes, nose, penis, ears.

3. Irrigation: NS or tap water, 50–100 mL/cm wound length, under pressure.

4. Debridement of devitalized tissue.

Closure:

1. Primary closure if clean, <12 hr old (extremity) or <24 hr (face/scalp).

2. Delayed closure for contaminated wounds, bites (except face), or crush injuries.

3. Leave puncture wounds open.

Tetanus prophylaxis:

1. Clean minor wound: Td/Tdap if >10 yrs since last dose.

2. All other wounds: Td/Tdap if >5 yrs since last dose.

3. Tetanus immune globulin (TIG) 250 U IM if uncertain/never immunized.

Antibiotics:

1. Dog/cat/human bites: Amoxicillin-clavulanate 875/125

mg PO BID × 5–7d (peds 22.5 mg/kg PO BID).

2. Penicillin allergy: Doxycycline 100 mg PO BID (peds >8 yrs) OR Clindamycin 10 mg/kg PO TID + Ciprofloxacin 20 mg/kg PO BID.

3. Open fractures: Cefazolin 2 g IV q8h (peds 30 mg/kg, max 2 g).

4. Gross contamination/farm injury: add Gentamicin 5 mg/kg IV.

5. Consider Rabies post-exposure prophylaxis for animal bites if risk.

WHEN TO CALL A SPECIALIST / TRANSFER

1. Open fractures.
2. Tendon, nerve, or vascular injury.
3. Grossly contaminated wounds needing operative washout.
4. Complex facial lacerations (cosmetic repair).
5. Hand bite wounds involving joints/tendons.

DISPOSITION

1. Discharge: simple wound repaired/cleaned, no red flags.
2. Admit locally: if IV antibiotics or observation needed.
3. Transfer: complex wounds, open fractures, vascular/tendon injury.

ADMISSION ORDERS (RURAL HOSPITAL)

1. Admit to monitored bed if IV antibiotics or observation

required.

2. Elevate affected limb, wound care with sterile dressings.

3. IV antibiotics as above.

4. Analgesia and tetanus prophylaxis.

5. Prepare for transfer if surgical management needed.

REFERENCES

1. Emergency Care BC — Wound Management: https://emergencycarebc.ca/clinical_resource

2. NICE CKS — Bites, Lacerations, Wound Care: https://cks.nice.org.uk

3. WHO — Wound and Trauma Care Guidance: https://www.who.int

4. CDC — Tetanus, Rabies & Wound Care Guidelines: https://www.cdc.gov

5. Canadian Paediatric Society — Bite Injuries and Wound Care: https://cps.ca

SECTION X – PEDIATRICS

PEDIATRIC FEVER (NEONATE VS CHILD) — RURAL ER APPROACH

OVERVIEW

Fever is one of the most common pediatric presentations in the rural ER. Etiologies range from benign viral infections to life-threatening bacterial sepsis or meningitis. Neonates (<28 days) are at highest risk for serious bacterial infection and require full sepsis evaluation. Children (1 month–16 years) require risk stratification based on age, appearance, and comorbidities. Rural priorities: stabilization, early sepsis recognition, empiric antibiotics when indicated, and transfer for high-risk cases.

CLINICAL PRESENTATION

Neonates (<28 days):
1. Often nonspecific: poor feeding, lethargy, irritability, apnea, hypothermia, or fever.
2. Fever ≥38.0°C (rectal) is always concerning.

Infants/Children:

1. Fever ± URI/GI symptoms, rash, ear pain, cough, sore throat.

2. May have signs of meningitis (neck stiffness, photophobia), pneumonia (tachypnea, retractions), or UTI (dysuria, frequency).

RED FLAGS

1. Neonates with any fever ≥38.0°C.

2. Toxic appearance, poor perfusion, shock.

3. Altered mental status, seizures.

4. Petechial or purpuric rash (meningococcemia).

5. Respiratory distress, SpO_2 <90%.

6. Immunocompromised child (chemo, steroids, sickle cell, asplenia).

DIFFERENTIAL DIAGNOSIS

1. Viral infections: influenza, RSV, adenovirus, COVID-19.

2. Bacterial infections: sepsis, meningitis, pneumonia, UTI, otitis media.

3. Inflammatory: Kawasaki disease, MIS-C (post COVID-19).

4. Non-infectious: malignancy, autoimmune disease, drug fever.

INVESTIGATIONS

Neonate (<28 days):

1. Full septic workup: CBC, electrolytes, blood culture, urine (catheter/suprapubic) with culture, LP for CSF.
2. CXR if respiratory symptoms.

Infants/Children:

1. Selective based on presentation.
2. CBC, blood culture if toxic.
3. Urinalysis/culture if <2 years with fever and no source.
4. CXR if tachypnea, hypoxemia, or focal findings.
5. LP if meningitis suspected.

MANAGEMENT IN RURAL ER (WITH DRUG DOSAGES)

General:

1. ABCs, oxygen as needed.
2. IV fluids: NS/LR 20 mL/kg bolus if shock.
3. Antipyretics: Acetaminophen 15 mg/kg PO/PR/ IV q6h (max 75 mg/kg/day). Ibuprofen 10 mg/kg PO q6–8h (if >6 months).

Neonate empiric antibiotics:

1. Ampicillin 50 mg/kg IV q6h + Gentamicin 5 mg/kg IV q24h.
2. Alternative: Ampicillin + Cefotaxime 50 mg/kg IV

q6–8h.

Infant/child empiric antibiotics (if toxic/septic):

1. Ceftriaxone 50 mg/kg IV/IM q24h (max 2 g).
2. Add Vancomycin 15 mg/kg IV q6h if meningitis or MRSA risk.

Seizure management (if febrile seizure):

1. Lorazepam 0.1 mg/kg IV (max 4 mg) or Midazolam 0.2 mg/kg intranasal/buccal.

WHEN TO CALL A SPECIALIST / TRANSFER

1. All neonates with fever.
2. Toxic-appearing children.
3. Suspected meningitis or sepsis.
4. Hemodynamic instability or respiratory failure.
5. Immunocompromised child with fever.
6. Failure to improve after resuscitation.

DISPOSITION

1. Discharge: only well-appearing child with clear viral source, reliable follow-up.
2. Admit locally: stable children with pneumonia, UTI, or dehydration manageable with IV therapy.
3. Transfer: all neonates, meningitis, sepsis, shock, unstable patients.

ADMISSION ORDERS (RURAL HOSPITAL)

1. Admit to monitored bed if indicated.
2. IV fluids, empiric antibiotics as above.
3. Antipyretics.
4. Strict I&O.
5. Neuro and cardiorespiratory monitoring.
6. Prepare transfer if unstable.

REFERENCES

1. Emergency Care BC — Pediatric Fever: https://emergencycarebc.ca/clinical_resource
2. NICE CKS — Fever in Under 5s: https://cks.nice.org.uk
3. WHO — Pocket Book of Hospital Care for Children: https://www.who.int
4. CDC — Pediatric Fever Guidance: https://www.cdc.gov
5. Canadian Paediatric Society — Fever and Infections in Children: https://cps.ca

PEDIATRIC RESPIRATORY DISTRESS (ASTHMA, BRONCHIOLITIS, CROUP) — RURAL ER APPROACH

OVERVIEW

Respiratory distress is one of the most common pediatric emergencies in the rural ER. Common causes include asthma exacerbations, bronchiolitis, and croup. Prompt recognition, supportive care, and appropriate pharmacologic interventions are critical to prevent respiratory failure. Rural priorities include early oxygen support, medication delivery, airway management if needed, and safe transfer for severe cases.

CLINICAL PRESENTATION

Asthma Exacerbation:
1. Wheezing, cough, chest tightness.
2. Tachypnea, accessory muscle use, hypoxemia.

Bronchiolitis (usually <2 years, RSV common):

1. Coryza, cough, tachypnea, wheezing, crackles.

2. Feeding difficulty, apnea in young infants.

Croup (laryngotracheitis, parainfluenza):

1. Barking cough, inspiratory stridor, hoarseness.

2. Worse at night, may present with respiratory distress.

RED FLAGS

1. SpO_2 <90% on room air.

2. Apnea, cyanosis.

3. Severe retractions, head bobbing, grunting.

4. Inability to feed or speak.

5. Lethargy, altered mental status.

6. Silent chest (severe asthma).

DIFFERENTIAL DIAGNOSIS

1. Asthma, bronchiolitis, croup.

2. Pneumonia.

3. Foreign body aspiration.

4. Anaphylaxis.

5. Congenital airway anomalies.

INVESTIGATIONS

Primarily clinical diagnosis.

Asthma:

1. Pulse oximetry.

2. CXR only if focal findings or severe.

Bronchiolitis:

1. Clinical diagnosis, CXR not routinely indicated.

Croup:

1. Clinical, no imaging needed unless atypical presentation.

MANAGEMENT IN RURAL ER (WITH DRUG DOSAGES)

General:

1. Oxygen to maintain SpO_2 ≥94%.
2. IV/IO access if severe.
3. Fluids for dehydration (caution in bronchiolitis).

Asthma Exacerbation:

1. Salbutamol: 2.5–5 mg nebulized q20 min ×3, then q1–4h PRN (peds 0.15 mg/kg/dose, max 5 mg).
2. Ipratropium: 250–500 mcg nebulized q20 min ×3 (peds 250 mcg).
3. Prednisone 1–2 mg/kg PO daily (max 50 mg) OR Dexamethasone 0.6 mg/kg PO/IV once (max 16 mg).
4. Magnesium sulfate 25–50 mg/kg IV over 20 min (max 2 g) for severe exacerbations.

Bronchiolitis:

1. Supportive: oxygen, nasal suction, hydration.
2. Trial of salbutamol may be considered if strong asthma

history.

3. No role for routine steroids/antibiotics.

Croup:

1. Dexamethasone 0.15–0.6 mg/kg PO/IM/IV once (max 16 mg).

2. Nebulized epinephrine (1:1000): 5 mL via nebulizer, repeat in 20 min if needed.

3. Observe at least 2 hours after epinephrine before discharge.

Adjuncts:

1. Antipyretics: Acetaminophen 15 mg/kg q6h (max 75 mg/kg/day).

WHEN TO CALL A SPECIALIST / TRANSFER

1. Severe distress unresponsive to initial therapy.

2. Requiring continuous nebulization or advanced airway support.

3. Apnea, cyanosis, altered LOC.

4. Infants <6 months with severe bronchiolitis.

5. Any child with persistent hypoxemia despite O_2.

DISPOSITION

1. Discharge: mild asthma or croup improved after treatment, stable bronchiolitis with good feeding.

2. Admit locally: moderate cases requiring O_2 or IV hydration.

3. Transfer: severe or refractory cases, need for ICU/ ventilation.

ADMISSION ORDERS (RURAL HOSPITAL)

1. Admit to monitored bed if persistent O_2 need.
2. Oxygen as needed.
3. Bronchodilator therapy for asthma.
4. IV fluids if unable to maintain oral intake.
5. Dexamethasone for croup, observe post-epinephrine.
6. Frequent vitals and SpO_2 monitoring.

REFERENCES

1. Emergency Care BC — Pediatric Asthma, Bronchiolitis, Croup: https://emergencycarebc.ca/ clinical_resource
2. NICE CKS — Asthma, Bronchiolitis, Croup in Children: https://cks.nice.org.uk
3. WHO — Pocket Book of Hospital Care for Children: https://www.who.int
4. CDC — Pediatric Respiratory Illness Guidance: https://www.cdc.gov
5. Canadian Paediatric Society — Acute Respiratory Conditions: https://cps.ca

PEDIATRIC SEIZURES & FEBRILE SEIZURES — RURAL ER APPROACH

OVERVIEW

Seizures are a common pediatric emergency and may be due to febrile illness, epilepsy, CNS infection, trauma, metabolic derangements, or toxins. Febrile seizures are the most common seizure type in children aged 6 months–5 years. They are usually benign but require differentiation from serious conditions such as meningitis. Rural ER priorities include airway protection, termination of seizure activity, investigation for underlying cause, and safe transfer if needed.

CLINICAL PRESENTATION

Generalized Seizures:
1. Tonic-clonic activity, loss of consciousness, post-ictal phase.
2. May present with incontinence, tongue biting.

Febrile Seizures:

1. Occur in children 6 months–5 years with fever ≥38°C.

2. Simple: generalized, <15 min, not recurrent in 24h, no neurologic deficit.

3. Complex: focal features, >15 min, recurrent within 24h, or post-ictal deficit.

Status Epilepticus:

1. Seizure lasting >5 minutes or recurrent seizures without recovery.

2. Life-threatening emergency requiring aggressive management.

RED FLAGS

1. Seizure >5 minutes (status epilepticus).

2. Focal seizure or post-ictal neurologic deficit.

3. Signs of meningitis or CNS infection.

4. Recurrent seizures without return to baseline.

5. Neonatal seizures (<1 month of age).

6. Persistent altered mental status.

DIFFERENTIAL DIAGNOSIS

1. Febrile seizure.

2. Epilepsy.

3. Meningitis/encephalitis.

4. Head trauma or intracranial hemorrhage.

5. Hypoglycemia, electrolyte disturbances (Na, Ca).

6. Toxic ingestion.

7. Breath-holding spells (benign).

INVESTIGATIONS

Bedside:

1. ABCs, glucose (fingerstick).
2. Vitals, SpO_2.

Labs:

1. CBC, electrolytes, calcium, magnesium, glucose.
2. Blood culture if febrile.

Other:

1. LP if meningitis suspected (do not delay antibiotics if unstable).
2. Neuroimaging (CT/MRI) if focal deficits, trauma, refractory seizures.

MANAGEMENT IN RURAL ER (WITH DRUG DOSAGES)

Immediate stabilization:

1. Airway: recovery position, suction, O_2.
2. IV/IO access, monitor.
3. Check glucose: give D10W 5 mL/kg IV if hypoglycemic.

Terminate seizure:

1. Lorazepam 0.1 mg/kg IV (max 4 mg) — may repeat once in 10 min.

2. If no IV: Midazolam 0.2 mg/kg IN/IM/buccal (max 10 mg).

3. Diazepam rectal gel 0.5 mg/kg if no IV/IN access (max 20 mg).

If persistent (>10–15 min):

1. Fosphenytoin 15–20 mg PE/kg IV at ≤1500 mg/min.

2. OR Phenytoin 15–20 mg/kg IV (max 1 g, infusion ≤50 mg/min).

3. Alternative: Levetiracetam 20–40 mg/kg IV (max 3 g).

Febrile seizure:

1. Simple: antipyretics, reassurance, no anticonvulsants needed.

2. Complex: manage as above + investigate underlying cause.

Adjuncts:

1. Antipyretics: Acetaminophen 15 mg/kg q6h (max 75 mg/kg/day); Ibuprofen 10 mg/kg q6–8h if >6 months.

WHEN TO CALL A SPECIALIST / TRANSFER

1. All status epilepticus or seizures >5 minutes.

2. Complex febrile seizures.

3. Any neonate with seizures.

4. Suspicion of CNS infection, trauma, or metabolic disorder.

5. Failure to return to baseline.

6. Any unstable child.

DISPOSITION

1. Discharge: simple febrile seizure, child well, reliable follow-up.
2. Admit locally: seizure with treatable cause (e.g., pneumonia, UTI) and stable.
3. Transfer: status epilepticus, neonatal seizure, complex febrile seizure, CNS infection.

ADMISSION ORDERS (RURAL HOSPITAL)

1. Admit to monitored bed if seizure cause unclear or ongoing risk.
2. IV access, seizure precautions.
3. Empiric antibiotics/antivirals if CNS infection suspected.
4. Antipyretics.
5. Frequent neuro checks and cardiorespiratory monitoring.

REFERENCES

1. Emergency Care BC — Seizures in Children: https://emergencycarebc.ca/clinical_resource
2. NICE CKS — Seizures, Epilepsy, Febrile Seizures: https://cks.nice.org.uk
3. WHO — Pocket Book of Hospital Care for Children: https://www.who.int
4. CDC — Pediatric Seizure & Epilepsy Guidance:

https://www.cdc.gov

5. Canadian Paediatric Society — Febrile Seizures
Practice Point: https://cps.ca

SECTION XI – OBSTETRICS & GYNECOLOGY

EARLY PREGNANCY EMERGENCIES (ECTOPIC, MISCARRIAGE) — RURAL ER APPROACH

OVERVIEW

Early pregnancy emergencies include ectopic pregnancy, threatened or spontaneous miscarriage, and septic abortion. These conditions are common in rural ER presentations and may be life-threatening due to hemorrhage or sepsis. Rural priorities include rapid diagnosis, hemodynamic stabilization, pain control, Rh immunoglobulin when indicated, and timely transfer to obstetrics/gynecology for definitive care.

CLINICAL PRESENTATION

Ectopic Pregnancy:
1. Abdominal/pelvic pain (often unilateral).
2. Vaginal bleeding.
3. Amenorrhea (4–10 weeks from LMP).

4.   Dizziness, syncope (if ruptured).

Miscarriage (threatened, inevitable, incomplete, complete, septic):

1.   Vaginal bleeding (light to heavy).

2.   Crampy lower abdominal pain.

3.   Passage of tissue.

4.   Fever, foul discharge (if septic).

RED FLAGS

1.   Hemodynamic instability (SBP <90, HR >120).

2.   Peritoneal signs (ruptured ectopic).

3.   Heavy vaginal bleeding (soaking >2 pads/hr).

4.   Fever, rigors, foul vaginal discharge (septic abortion).

5.   Severe anemia or shock.

DIFFERENTIAL DIAGNOSIS

1.   Ectopic pregnancy.

2.   Threatened/incomplete miscarriage.

3.   Complete miscarriage.

4.   Molar pregnancy.

5.   Pelvic inflammatory disease.

6.   Non-gynecologic: appendicitis, renal colic.

INVESTIGATIONS

Bedside:

1. Vitals, urine pregnancy test.

2. POCUS: intrauterine vs ectopic pregnancy, free fluid.

Labs:

1. Quantitative β-hCG.

2. CBC, electrolytes, renal function.

3. Blood type & screen (Rh status).

4. Blood cultures if septic abortion suspected.

MANAGEMENT IN RURAL ER (WITH DRUG DOSAGES)

General stabilization:

1. Oxygen, IV fluids (NS/LR bolus 1–2 L adults).

2. Analgesia: Morphine 2–5 mg IV q2–4h PRN (peds 0.05–0.1 mg/kg).

3. Antiemetics: Ondansetron 4 mg IV q6–8h.

Ectopic Pregnancy (suspected/confirmed):

1. NPO, IV access ×2 large bore.

2. Prepare for urgent transfer if unstable.

3. Do NOT give methotrexate in ER — requires specialist assessment.

Miscarriage:

1. Threatened: observe, pelvic rest, outpatient follow-up if stable.

2. Incomplete/inevitable: IV fluids, pain control, prepare transfer for evacuation.

3. Septic abortion: start broad-spectrum antibiotics immediately:
   - • - Piperacillin–Tazobactam 4.5 g IV q6h (peds 80 mg/kg q6h, max 4.5 g).
   - • - OR Clindamycin 900 mg IV q8h + Gentamicin 5–7 mg/kg IV daily.

Rh Prophylaxis:

1. If Rh-negative and <20 weeks: Rh immunoglobulin 50 mcg IM once.
2. If ≥20 weeks: Rh immunoglobulin 300 mcg IM once.

WHEN TO CALL A SPECIALIST / TRANSFER

1. All suspected ectopic pregnancies.
2. Hemodynamically unstable patients.
3. Septic abortion.
4. Heavy or persistent bleeding.
5. Need for surgical evacuation or transfusion.

DISPOSITION

1. Discharge: threatened miscarriage only, stable, with reliable follow-up.
2. Admit locally: only if mild and awaiting transfer.
3. Transfer: ectopic pregnancy, incomplete/septic abortion, unstable bleeding.

ADMISSION ORDERS (RURAL HOSPITAL)

1. Admit to monitored bed if unstable and awaiting

transfer.

2. Oxygen, IV fluids.

3. Broad-spectrum antibiotics if septic abortion.

4. Pain control and antiemetics.

5. Rh immunoglobulin if indicated.

6. Monitor vitals q15–30 min.

REFERENCES

1. Emergency Care BC — Early Pregnancy Emergencies: https://emergencycarebc.ca/clinical_resource

2. NICE CKS — Ectopic Pregnancy & Miscarriage: https://cks.nice.org.uk

3. Canadian Paediatric Society — Reproductive Emergencies: https://cps.ca

4. CDC — Reproductive Health Guidance: https://www.cdc.gov

5. WHO — Maternal Health & Abortion Care Guidelines: https://www.who.int

THIRD-TRIMESTER EMERGENCIES (PRE-ECLAMPSIA, ECLAMPSIA, PLACENTAL ABRUPTION) — RURAL ER APPROACH

OVERVIEW

Third-trimester emergencies such as pre-eclampsia, eclampsia, and placental abruption are leading causes of maternal and fetal morbidity and mortality. In rural ERs, priorities include early recognition, stabilization, seizure prevention/control, blood pressure management, maternal resuscitation, fetal monitoring if possible, and urgent transfer to obstetrics/tertiary care.

- - Pre-eclampsia: new hypertension + proteinuria or end-organ dysfunction after 20 weeks.
- - Eclampsia: pre-eclampsia complicated by seizures.
- - Placental Abruption: premature separation of placenta causing maternal hemorrhage and fetal distress.

CLINICAL PRESENTATION

Pre-eclampsia:

1. BP ≥140/90 after 20 weeks + proteinuria (>300 mg/24h) or symptoms.
2. Headache, visual changes, RUQ/epigastric pain, edema.

Eclampsia:

1. Generalized tonic-clonic seizures.
2. May occur before, during, or after delivery.

Placental Abruption:

1. Vaginal bleeding (may be concealed).
2. Sudden abdominal/back pain, uterine tenderness, board-like uterus.
3. Fetal distress or absent fetal heart tones.
4. Maternal shock out of proportion to visible blood loss.

RED FLAGS

1. Severe hypertension: SBP ≥160 or DBP ≥110 mmHg.
2. Visual changes, severe headache, altered mental status.
3. Seizures.
4. Oliguria, pulmonary edema, rising creatinine.
5. Fetal distress or absent fetal movement.
6. Hypotension, tachycardia, shock (placental

abruption).

DIFFERENTIAL DIAGNOSIS

1. Gestational hypertension without proteinuria.

2. Epilepsy, hypoglycemia, stroke (for seizures).

3. Placenta previa, uterine rupture (for bleeding).

4. Appendicitis, cholecystitis, renal colic (non-OB abdominal pain).

INVESTIGATIONS

Bedside:

1. Vitals, SpO_2, urine dip for protein.

2. Bedside fetal heart tones if Doppler available.

Labs:

1. CBC, electrolytes, creatinine, LFTs, coagulation profile.

2. Type & crossmatch.

Imaging:

1. Ultrasound (if available): assess fetus, placenta, rule out previa.

2. Definitive diagnosis of abruption is clinical.

MANAGEMENT IN RURAL ER (WITH DRUG DOSAGES)

General stabilization:

1. Oxygen, 2 large-bore IV lines.

2. IV fluids: NS/LR bolus 1 L, titrate to avoid overload.

3. Monitor maternal and fetal status.

Pre-eclampsia/Eclampsia:

1. Seizure prophylaxis/treatment: Magnesium sulfate 4 g IV over 20 min, then 1 g/hr IV infusion. (Peds: not typically used).

2. If seizure recurs: additional $MgSO_4$ 2 g IV over 5–10 min.

3. Antidote if magnesium toxicity: Calcium gluconate 10 mL of 10% IV over 10 min.

4. Antihypertensives: Labetalol 20 mg IV over 2 min, then 40 mg after 10 min if needed (max 220 mg); OR Hydralazine 5–10 mg IV q20–30 min (max 30 mg).

5. Nifedipine 10 mg PO may be used if IV access limited.

Placental Abruption:

1. Resuscitation with fluids, blood if available.

2. Oxygen, left lateral position.

3. Monitor urine output with Foley.

4. Avoid tocolytics.

5. Prepare for emergent transfer.

WHEN TO CALL A SPECIALIST / TRANSFER

1. All suspected eclampsia or abruption.

2. Severe pre-eclampsia (SBP ≥160/DBP ≥110, symptoms).

3. Maternal hemodynamic instability.

4. Fetal distress or intrauterine demise.

5. Arrange urgent transfer to obstetrics/tertiary care center.

DISPOSITION

1. Discharge: not appropriate.

2. Admit locally: only if awaiting transfer and stable.

3. Transfer urgently for definitive management.

ADMISSION ORDERS (RURAL HOSPITAL)

1. Admit to monitored bed while awaiting transfer.

2. Oxygen, IV fluids, seizure precautions.

3. Magnesium sulfate infusion.

4. Antihypertensives as above.

5. Foley catheter, strict I&O.

6. Serial vitals and neuro checks.

7. Prepare blood products if available.

REFERENCES

1. Emergency Care BC — Pre-eclampsia/Eclampsia & Obstetric Emergencies: https://emergencycarebc.ca/clinical_resource

2. NICE CKS — Hypertension in Pregnancy: https://cks.nice.org.uk

3. WHO — Maternal Health Guidelines: https://www.who.int

4. CDC — Pregnancy-Related Health Guidance: https://

www.cdc.gov

5. Canadian Paediatric Society — Perinatal Emergencies: https://cps.ca

NORMAL DELIVERY IN THE ER (PRECIPITOUS BIRTH, SHOULDER DYSTOCIA, POSTPARTUM HEMORRHAGE) — RURAL ER APPROACH

OVERVIEW

In rural ERs, unplanned deliveries may occur before transfer to obstetrics. Complications include precipitous birth, shoulder dystocia, and postpartum hemorrhage (PPH). These require rapid recognition, structured management, and preparation for neonatal resuscitation. Rural priorities include safe delivery technique, maternal stabilization, uterotonic therapy, and transfer if complications arise.

CLINICAL PRESENTATION

Precipitous Birth:
1. Rapid labor and delivery (<3 hours).
2. May be associated with perineal tears, PPH.

Shoulder Dystocia:

1. Fetal head delivers but anterior shoulder is stuck behind pubic symphysis.
2. 'Turtle sign' (retraction of head).

Postpartum Hemorrhage:

1. Bleeding >500 mL after vaginal birth or >1000 mL after C-section.
2. Uterine atony most common cause.
3. May also result from trauma, retained tissue, or coagulopathy.

RED FLAGS

1. Uncontrolled bleeding after delivery.
2. Failure to deliver shoulders after head (shoulder dystocia).
3. Hypotension, tachycardia, shock in mother.
4. Neonatal distress (poor tone, color, cry, or HR <100 bpm).

DIFFERENTIAL DIAGNOSIS

1. Vaginal bleeding due to laceration or uterine rupture.
2. Retained placenta or products of conception.
3. Neonatal asphyxia (cord prolapse, shoulder dystocia).

INVESTIGATIONS

Primarily a clinical diagnosis and emergency management.

If stable:

1. CBC, coagulation, type and crossmatch.

2. Bedside ultrasound: retained products, uterine tone.

3. Neonatal: APGAR assessment, bedside glucose if poor condition.

MANAGEMENT IN RURAL ER (WITH DRUG DOSAGES)

Precipitous Birth:

1. Support perineum, control head delivery.

2. Suction mouth then nose if obstructed.

3. Dry, stimulate newborn, assess with APGAR.

4. Clamp and cut cord after 30–60 sec.

Shoulder Dystocia:

1. Call for help, note time of head delivery.

2. McRoberts maneuver: hyperflex maternal hips.

3. Suprapubic pressure (NOT fundal pressure).

4. Delivery of posterior arm if unsuccessful.

5. Consider all-fours position if persistent.

Postpartum Hemorrhage (Uterine Atony):

1. Uterine massage.

2. Oxytocin: 10 IU IM once, OR 20–40 IU in 1 L NS/LR at 125 mL/hr IV infusion.

3. Misoprostol: 800–1000 mcg PR once.

4. Carboprost (Hemabate): 250 mcg IM q15–20 min (max

2 mg) [avoid in asthma].

5. Tranexamic acid: 1 g IV over 10 min, repeat after 30 min if needed.

6. Replace fluids, blood as available.

General:

1. Foley catheter, monitor urine output.

2. Oxygen, IV fluids.

3. Neonatal resuscitation if indicated: PPV with bag-mask if HR <100 bpm.

4. Prepare transfer if ongoing PPH or neonatal compromise.

WHEN TO CALL A SPECIALIST / TRANSFER

1. All cases of shoulder dystocia.

2. Ongoing PPH despite uterotonics.

3. Severe perineal lacerations.

4. Neonatal resuscitation beyond basic steps.

5. Urgent transfer if mother unstable or neonate compromised.

DISPOSITION

1. Discharge: only if uncomplicated delivery, mother stable, neonate well, and safe follow-up.

2. Admit locally: if mild PPH controlled and both mother and neonate stable.

3. Transfer: all complicated cases (shoulder dystocia, uncontrolled PPH, neonatal compromise).

ADMISSION ORDERS (RURAL HOSPITAL)

1. Admit to monitored bed if postpartum complication.
2. Oxytocin infusion as above.
3. Monitor vitals, bleeding, urine output.
4. CBC, coagulation, crossmatch.
5. Neonatal monitoring: vitals, glucose, feeding support.
6. Prepare for transfer if unstable.

REFERENCES

1. Emergency Care BC — Obstetric Emergencies: https://emergencycarebc.ca/clinical_resource
2. NICE CKS — Labour & Delivery Complications: https://cks.nice.org.uk
3. WHO — Maternal & Newborn Care Guidelines: https://www.who.int
4. CDC — Pregnancy & Delivery Guidance: https://www.cdc.gov
5. Canadian Paediatric Society — Neonatal Resuscitation: https://cps.ca

VAGINAL BLEEDING & VAGINITIS — RURAL ER APPROACH

OVERVIEW

Vaginal bleeding and vaginitis are common presentations in the rural ER. Bleeding may be due to benign causes (dysfunctional uterine bleeding, fibroids, polyps), early pregnancy complications, or malignancy. Vaginitis is often infectious (bacterial vaginosis, Candida, Trichomonas) but may also be due to atrophic or irritant causes. The rural ER role is stabilization, initial management, symptom relief, and referral for definitive care.

CLINICAL PRESENTATION

Vaginal Bleeding:
1. Heavy menstrual bleeding, intermenstrual bleeding, postmenopausal bleeding.
2. May present with anemia, hemodynamic instability.
3. In pregnancy: threatened miscarriage, ectopic, placenta previa, abruption.

Vaginitis:

1. Vaginal discharge, odor, pruritus, dysuria, dyspareunia.

2. BV: thin gray discharge, fishy odor.

3. Candida: thick white 'cottage cheese' discharge, vulvar itching.

4. Trichomonas: frothy yellow-green discharge, strawberry cervix.

RED FLAGS

1. Hemodynamic instability with vaginal bleeding.

2. Postmenopausal bleeding (consider malignancy).

3. Pregnancy with bleeding and pain.

4. Severe vulvar pain, necrosis, systemic toxicity (necrotizing infection).

5. Recurrent or persistent vaginitis despite treatment.

DIFFERENTIAL DIAGNOSIS

1. Abnormal uterine bleeding (fibroids, polyps, anovulation).

2. Early pregnancy complications.

3. Vaginitis: BV, Candida, Trichomonas.

4. STIs: chlamydia, gonorrhea, herpes.

5. Atrophic vaginitis (postmenopausal).

INVESTIGATIONS

Bedside:

1. Vitals, pregnancy test (urine/serum β-hCG).

2. Speculum exam: bleeding source, discharge, cervix.

Labs:

1. CBC, coagulation profile if heavy bleeding.

2. Vaginal swabs for microscopy/culture/NAAT.

3. STI screening (chlamydia, gonorrhea, syphilis, HIV).

Imaging:

1. Pelvic ultrasound if available (structural causes, retained tissue, adnexal masses).

MANAGEMENT IN RURAL ER (WITH DRUG DOSAGES)

Vaginal Bleeding:

1. Stabilize if heavy bleeding: oxygen, IV fluids (NS/LR 1–2 L bolus).

2. Tranexamic acid 1 g IV over 10 min, may repeat in 30 min (peds: 15 mg/kg, max 1 g/dose).

3. Consider high-dose hormonal therapy (if non-pregnant, not contraindicated): Combined OCPs (ethinyl estradiol 30–35 mcg + progestin, 1 tab PO TID × 7 days).

4. Iron supplementation if anemic.

Vaginitis (Empiric options):

1. Bacterial Vaginosis: Metronidazole 500 mg PO BID × 7 days.

2. Candidiasis: Fluconazole 150 mg PO single dose; OR Clotrimazole 500 mg PV single dose.

3. Trichomoniasis: Metronidazole 2 g PO single dose (treat partner as well).

Adjuncts:

1. Analgesia: Acetaminophen 650–1000 mg PO q6h (peds 15 mg/kg q6h).

2. Avoid vaginal douching or irritants.

3. STI counseling and safe sex education.

WHEN TO CALL A SPECIALIST / TRANSFER

1. Hemodynamic instability, transfusion requirement.

2. Suspected ectopic pregnancy or obstetric cause.

3. Postmenopausal bleeding (rule out malignancy).

4. Recurrent or refractory vaginitis.

5. Necrotizing infection or severe systemic illness.

DISPOSITION

1. Discharge: stable, mild bleeding, uncomplicated vaginitis with follow-up.

2. Admit locally: moderate bleeding needing observation, IV fluids, or blood.

3. Transfer: unstable hemorrhage, obstetric emergencies, suspected malignancy needing urgent workup.

ADMISSION ORDERS (RURAL HOSPITAL)

1. Admit to monitored bed if unstable bleeding.
2. IV fluids, blood transfusion if available.
3. Tranexamic acid as above.
4. CBC, coagulation monitoring.
5. Empiric vaginitis therapy if appropriate.
6. Arrange urgent follow-up with gynecology.

REFERENCES

1. Emergency Care BC — Vaginal Bleeding & Vaginitis: https://emergencycarebc.ca/clinical_resource
2. NICE CKS — Vaginal Discharge, Abnormal Uterine Bleeding: https://cks.nice.org.uk
3. WHO — Reproductive Health Guidelines: https://www.who.int
4. CDC — STI & Vaginitis Treatment Guidelines: https://www.cdc.gov
5. Canadian Paediatric Society — Adolescent Gynecology: https://cps.ca